Plato's Barbell

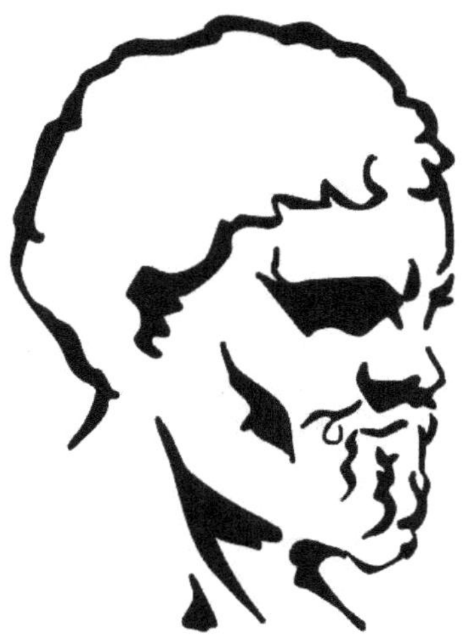

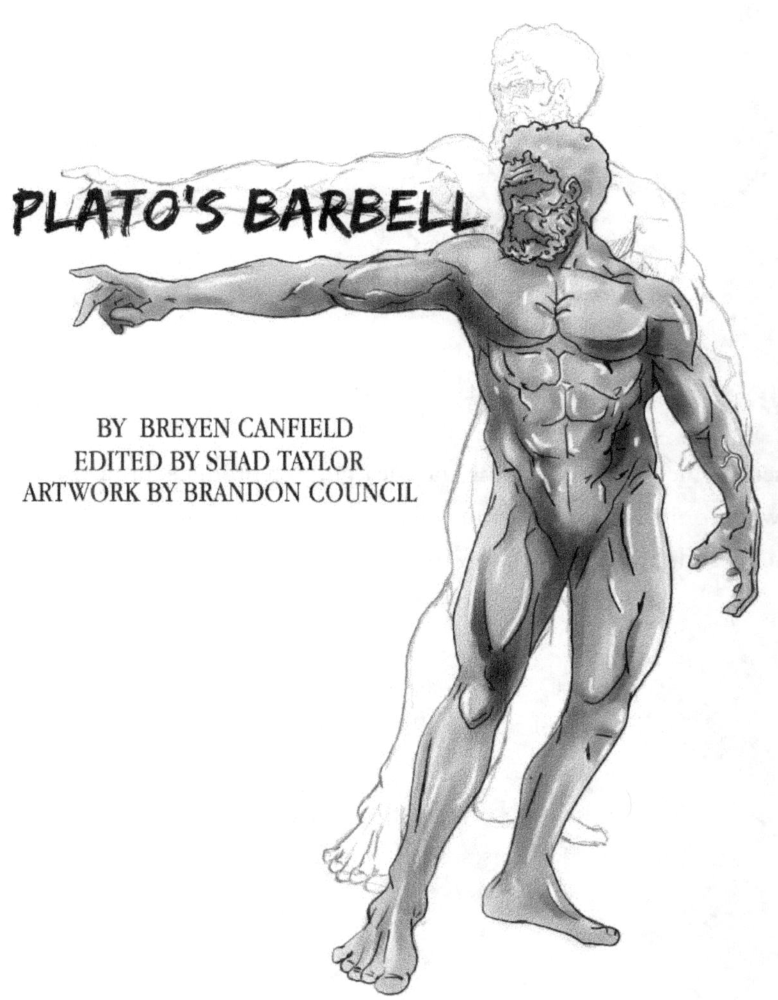

PLATO'S BARBELL

BY BREYEN CANFIELD
EDITED BY SHAD TAYLOR
ARTWORK BY BRANDON COUNCIL

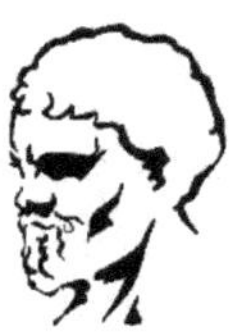

Copyright © 2023

Plato's Barbell
platosbarbell.com

Published by Jailhouse Strong
jailhousestrong.com

For The Dude, Val Balison.
Special thanks to Billy Bybee and Michael and Joshua Baumgarten.
Katie, David, Avery, and Jack: thank you for your patience. I love you.

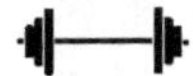

Plato's Barbell

Contents

Introduction

In *How Architecture Works* Witold Rybczynski writes "ultimately, we recognize the spirit of architecture in any building that exhibits a coherent visual language." The architect and professor then quotes modernist architecture pioneer Mies van der Rohe's observation that "architecture starts when you carefully put two bricks together."

Why introduce a book about philosophy and weightlifting with architecture quotes? If the parallels between philosophy and weightlifting are not immediately obvious then the parallels between philosophy and weightlifting and architecture are probably less so. But further investigation reveals a helpful conveyance of the bridges between form and function, aesthetics and performance and—most fundamental to our conversation—efficient approaches to closing the gap between all of the above.

Our attempt to analogize architecture and weightlifting crumbles slightly when Rybczynski seems to lament that "exactly what makes a building memorable is hard to pin down." Fans of weightlifting might fondly recall Naim Süleymanoğlu's 190kg clean and jerk at the 1988 Olympic Games in Seoul, South Korea, Mattias Steiner's 258kg clean and jerk to win gold at the 2008 Olympic Games in Beijing, China following his wife's death in 2007, or Kakhi Kakhiashvili's world record setting 235kg clean and jerk to tie Sergei

Syrtsov's 412.5kg total, allowing Kakhiashvili to top the podium in Barcelona, Spain at the 1992 Olympic Games due to the Georgian's bodyweight tiebreaker advantage over his Unified Teammate, who hailed from Russia. New fans of the sport may be curious why all of the listed moments feature clean and jerks with no snatches. The fact that the clean and jerk follows the snatch in Olympic style competitions lends it a sort of recency bias in our memories of these glorious moments. Andrei Rybakou's 187kg snatch at the 2007 World Championships in Chiang Mai, Thailand, Andrei Aramnau's 200kg snatch at the 2008 Olympics in Beijing, China, and Lasha Talakhadze's first 220kg snatch at the World Championships in Anaheim, California all make that list of memorable lifts and would likely be interchangeable if the snatch and clean and jerk's order were reversed in competition formats.

But—an astute reader might say to herself—these all seem to be lifts that won medals and could therefore be considered memorable *moments* rather than memorable *lifts*. Like most athletic achievements across all sports, what makes a lift memorable *as a moment* is that that lift is precisely what is required *in that moment* and that is what makes it memorable. Plenty of medals, trophies, cups, and other memorabilia are won in all levels of competition that no one other than the lifter and her coach will remember. At the highest level of competition, however, the sport reaches its peak both in magnitude and performance; more viewers tune in to watch the Olympic Games—however difficult television production teams insist on making tuning in—than tune in to watch whatever local meet might be happening in a high school gymnasium on any given Saturday. This, then, is why Rybczynski's commentary on a building's memorability runs adrift our attempt to discuss weightlifting on architecture's terms: a building in some time and space could be any building, but a snatch or clean and jerk in the time and space we mentioned could hardly have been any other lift.

If Rybakou's left foot had slipped when walking the overhead bar forward that first step, then that 187kg world record snatch would not have occurred, and no one would consider it one of history's great lifts. If

Süleymanoğlu hadn't wiggled his hips from stage left to stage right with just the right amount of pressure, the 190kg resting uncomfortably in his front rack position likely would have fallen to its more appropriate resting place on the platform below. Unlike a building, which could really be any forgettable building at any place in any moment, only these movements could move these weights above these lifters' heads. Returning to our analogy, even though the professor tells us that "most architecture is experienced in bits and pieces," and that appreciation of architecture is sometimes appreciation of little more than "just a detail," that detail is enough to make us nod and acknowledge "how nice" it is that "someone actually thought of that." For Rybczynski, in building and buildings "that" might be a "well-shaped door handle, a window framing a perfect little view, a rosette carved into a chapel pew." For our weightlifter, or a fan of the sport, the "that" might be a well-placed toe, maintenance of a vertical torso, or a perfectly timed dip and drive between oscillations of a plated barbell between a clean and a jerk. These appreciations might be minute or appreciated almost solely by the most deeply initiated while that which frustrates the same sort of individual is much more basic, if no more obvious to the uninitiated; a point that brings these parallels full circle and underscores Rybczynski's final admonition:

> *"As someone who has practiced architecture, I find it difficult to excuse technical incompetence in the name of experimentation, or to overlook functional deficiencies for the sake of artistic purity. Architecture is an applied art, and it is in the application that the architect often finds inspiration. I confess to a partiality for those who face this challenge squarely, rather than withdraw to hermetic theories or personal quests."*

What, then, are we supposed to take from this introduction? First that—while weightlifting and buildings may not be exactly analogous—a lifter's movement through time and space requires thoughtful construction much like that of a church, museum, or other historically memorable building. Second, this movement construction begins immediately when the two bricks of the athlete and the barbell are rubbed together. Third, while all of the pieces of a movement might be experienced in bits and pieces and thus may necessarily be trained that way, none of them function properly without the others in their proper place. Finally, while artistic expression and beauty of the movement are important to the lifts, that expression of beauty is only necessary because of the efficiency they lend to the movement. And, like the professor and architect says, it is difficult to excuse a lack of technical competence at the expense of artistic purity and those who pursue the latter must first master the former.

And for the tie-in between architecture and weightlifting and philosophy and weightlifting? Now that we have spent a little time considering the themes common to two undertakings as categorically distinct as weightlifting and architecture, investigating the themes common to one of the most physically violent movements on one side and one of history's most thoughtfully academic pastimes on the other side may be less overwhelming. Or at least less brow-furrowing to weightlifters, philosophers, and—probably most common—those of us who fall somewhere in between.

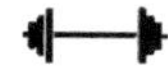

Preface

While this book is called *Plato's Barbell,* we rely on many more philosophers to build our understanding of coaching, learning, and moving. Plato, 428 BC - 347 BC, is credited with writing dozens of works, almost entirely in dialogue form. Most of these dialogues feature a central character familiar to most anyone who has read, studied, or even simply heard of philosophy: Socrates. Through Socrates and his dialectic partners Plato investigates beauty, justice, the nature of reality, and humankind's role in the universe. These investigations are fundamental to Plato's role in the creation of the academy, the predecessor to modern universities. Over two thousand years after Plato's death, philosophy professor and mathematician, Alfred North Whitehead, summarized the entire catalog of western philosophy calling it "a series of footnotes to Plato." As with most footnotes the philosophers and the philosophies we analyze in this book serve to clarify or expound concepts that can likely be traced all the way back to the Athenian.

In addition to his writings on social and political philosophy and ethics and morals, Plato—through his Socratic dialogues—proposed the idea that there is some eternal, perfect realm in which *Forms* exist. In the world in which we live we only observe imperfect objects that participate in the likeness of the perfect forms. For Plato a barbell is a tool we can use to perform a snatch or a clean and jerk, but that barbell is imperfect because it will one day degrade and cease to exist. However, even if all barbells in space and time cease to exist, the *Form* or *Idea* of a barbell is eternal. Better or worse barbells can participate more or less perfectly or imperfectly in the form or idea of a barbell, but Plato's Theory of Forms provides us a tool to get closer to not only the ideal barbell, but the ideal snatch, clean and jerk, and all other movements that supplement Olympic weightlifting.

A few hundred years after Plato wrote, a Greek named Epictetus worked to apply many of the more theoretical aspects of Stoicism; a school of thought founded by Zeno of Citium in the 3rd century BC. For Epictetus, a former slave educated under a Roman senator after being freed, philosophy was more than an academic exercise. Inspired by Socrates, whose dialectics Epictetus quotes frequently throughout his *Discourses*, the former slave focuses much of his attention applying the questions of philosophy to everyday life. Epictetus asked one of his most fundamental questions in Chapter XI of Book II of his *Discourses*, "What is the Beginning of Philosophy?" What Epictetus finds shows the value of philosophy for those who practice it *the right way*.

Just as no one walks into a gym knowing the proper way to snatch, clean, or even front or back squat, Epictetus reminds us that no one is born with proper conceptions of right-angled triangles, or musical tones or semitones. There are, however, some ideas that we do not need to learn about in order to know of them. All rational people are born with some innate sense of right and wrong, good and bad, happiness and unhappiness, and many other concepts that Epictetus categorizes as personal opinion. Where there is no tension surrounding inquiry into whether a triangle is a right-angled triangle, nor whether a barbell lifted from the floor directly overhead without pausing on the front rack of the shoulders is a snatch and not a clean and jerk, there is likely to be tension when one person applies her conception of *good* to a proposition another person applies his conception of *good* to when what is good and bad means something different to each of them. Here, says Epictetus, we see the beginning of philosophy:

> *...in the discovery of the conflict of men's minds with one another, and the attempt to seek for the reason of this conflict, and the condemnation of mere opinion, as a thing not to be trusted; and a search to determine whether your opinion is true, and an attempt to discover a standard, just as we discover the balance to deal with weights and the rule to deal with things straight and crooked. This is the beginning of philosophy.[1]*

There is no question what constitutes a made or missed lift. But judges can be right or wrong about whether an individual lift was made or missed. There is likewise no question what a back squat is and what a deadlift is. But there are numerous evaluations whether an individual back squat or deadlift is better or worse than any other individual back squat or deadlift. Going back to Plato, we can more easily determine what the perfect *Form* of a movement is: a snatch must feature a single fluid movement of the barbell from the floor to the overhead position without coming to rest at any point and without being pressed out by the lifter's arms. Any observable snatch that fails to participate in this *Form* of the snatch will—or at least should—be judged a missed lift. But where Plato is concerned with an observable movement's participation in its perfect form, Epictetus is concerned with resolving the tension between the evaluations of the made or missed lifts and the better or worse back squats or deadlifts.

What each judge or observer thinks is important to getting us nearer a conception of the best version of each lift but "what each man thinks," Epictetus tells us, "is not sufficient to make a thing so." Once we find some agreed upon standard, he goes on, discovery of that agreed upon standard "relieves from madness those who wrongly use personal opinion as their only measure, and enables us thereafter to start from known principles, clearly defined." Once the judge or observer begins working from a set of known and clearly defined principles, each is able to apply her conception to particular instances in "definite and articulate form."[2]

Epictetus does not tell us exactly how to get each judge or observer to agree on any set of known and clearly defined principles, but that is not what he is trying to do. Similarly, this book is not an attempt to track down precisely the optimal application of leverage, moment and lever arm, and technically proficient application of force necessary to lift world record shattering weights. This book is an attempt to use philosophy to discover the right way to learn, practice, and perfect weightlifting beyond mere opinion.

There are going to be as many approaches to this task as there are men and women contemplating the right approach. How, then, should we measure the rightness of the approach? As the approach that works for the best lifter? Or the approach that works best for the most lifters? Maybe there is more than one right approach; more than one approach known, clearly defined, and accepted by many or all readers. But maybe we are asking the wrong questions when we ask what the *right* approach is.

At the end of the day, the bar goes up and the bar goes down. The judge's lights are either white or red, the medals gold, silver, or bronze. Are those not the sort of judgements and measurements Epictetus says we should use to get past mere opinion in order to more agreeably decide whether a thing is good or bad or right or wrong? Closer to or further from Plato's *Forms*? In Epictetus's own words: "thus things are judged and weighed if we have standards ready to test them: and in fact the work of philosophy is to investigate and firmly establish such standards; and the duty of the good man is to proceed to apply the decisions arrived at."

This is the beginning of philosophy.

This is Plato's Barbell.[3]

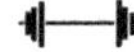

On Perfection: Platonism and Competition

There are two immediately obvious types of competition: competition against the other, and competition against the self. Competition against the other is clearly definable as at least one competitor performing some skill or set of skills against another competitor or group of other competitors. Competition against the self, however, is probably more accurately described as an attempt at perfection of the self. Some exceptionally gifted competitors may possess a set of natural talents that allows them to win some competition against others while performing far below a level of performance of which they are personally capable. This talent may be enough to permit the competitor to win a competition against another seemingly without putting in any work, or the talent may be a capacity for work that lets that competitor sharpen and strengthen the skill sets necessary to win such a competition. This is not to say that these world beating competitors do not also compete against themselves; only that the level of competition against others does not rise to the level of competition of which they are capable, i.e., their potential level of competition against the self is a higher level than that of the necessary level of competition against the other. Some other competitors may not possess such a set of natural talents and instead compete with themselves either in an effort to raise the level of their own performance for its own sake, or to improve the level of their own performance in order to improve their chances to win a competition against some other competitor.

In each case, the ultimate end of competition—either against the other or the self—is to be the best: to outperform one's rival and stand atop the podium, whether the lower podium steps hold other competitors or inferior executions of one's own prior performances. However, despite having a clear and defined goal, in each case *the best* is somewhat ambiguously defined. More crucially, even if that definition is clear, which goal is preferable is still in contention. Is it better for a coach to create a methodology based on simply helping her athlete beat some other athlete in a given competition? Or is it better for a coach to create a methodology focused solely on perfecting her athlete's ability to perform? Finally, is there even a difference between these two approaches? Answering these questions will render these incompatible versions of the term best relatively unimportant; deciding which methodology a coach should focus on will take care of the rest.

For Plato, there are two worlds: the world of the Forms and the physical world in which Forms are represented.[4] The Form of some thing is the abstract, perfect, idealized version of some thing's observable, imperfect, instantiated form In his introduction to Plato's *Complete Works*, John M. Cooper describes Plato's Forms as "eternal, nonphysical, quintessentially unitary entities, knowledge of which is attainable by abstract and theoretical thought, standing immutably in the nature of things as standards on which the physical world and the world of moral relationships among human beings are themselves grounded." If there is some thing that we can see, hear, feel, or somehow otherwise measure here on Earth, Plato teaches that there is a perfect version of it in the realm of the Forms.[5] It is this Form in which all sensible versions share some of the Form's quality and that quality is what makes them that thing.[6] So long as a sensible version of some thing emulates its Formal version, that sensible thing is recognizable and usable, at least as that thing is intended. As Socrates says, "when a craftsman discovers the type of tool that is naturally suited for a given type of work, he must embody it in the material out of which he is making the tool."[7] He goes on to suggest that for a blacksmith attempting to forge a drill out of iron, "as long as they give it the same form—even if that form is embodied in different iron—the tool will be correct, whether it is made in Greece or abroad."[8]

Furthermore, the Forms are perfect, unlike any potential sensible instantiation of any Form.[9] When a cabinetmaker picks up a saw and a plane, it is unlikely that she is setting out to make an imperfect cabinet. She likely has some idea in her head about what a perfect cabinet is. Another cabinetmaker in another shop may pick up his own saw and plane and attempt to make his version of a perfect cabinet. It does not matter that their finished cabinets will almost certainly come out differently, only that they share enough of the Platonic Form of a cabinet that a non-cabinetmaker will be able to see the finished products and identify the products as some sort of storage container. The Form of a cabinet is the perfect version all cabinetmakers attempt to emulate, whether or not they have read 5th century BC Greek philosophy. Without this perfect Form, there is no way to differentiate from a better or worse cabinet. Perhaps one supposed cabinet is more beautiful, but it has no storage; it could hardly be considered a cabinet at all if it cannot be used to store anything. Without some shared sense of what everyone considers a cabinet, there would be no objective standard by which to measure cabit*ness*. That sense of a thing's *-ness*, the one we all share when contemplating any sensible thing, is its Platonic Form.

We can even extrapolate that it is the ability to grasp that which resides in the realm of the Forms with true knowledge.[10] Plato's theory, that what we can observe is merely a set of representations of that which is perfect in the realm of the Forms, is further augmented in his Allegory of the Cave. In his *Republic* Plato illustrates that most of us are living in a cave and everything we see is just a shadow on a wall; silhouettes of images held up by puppeteers standing in front of a fire.[11] It is only when we break free of the shackles that bind us to the cave that we are able to turn "the whole soul until it is able to study that which is and the brightest thing that is, namely, the one we call the good."[12] There is nothing about this journey that is easy. Along the way, the cave dweller will face distractions, confusion, and temptation to revert back to his cave-dwelling ways. However, once one is able to focus on that which is perfect, the Forms, and not the mere images that line the cave walls, one becomes able to embrace the "virtue of reason" which "seems to belong above all to something more divine, which never loses its power but is either useful and beneficial or useless and harmful, depending on the way it is turned."[13]

Plato tells us "that the ones who get to this point are unwilling to occupy themselves with human affairs and that their souls are always pressing upwards, eager to spend their time above."[14] It is illogical, then, to believe that concerning oneself with the affairs of others can ever provide a path toward true perfection. Arguably, for Plato, perfection is the path itself.

So what about the seemingly incompatible theories of competition? What does Plato have to offer a coach—and by extension an athlete—seeking a spot atop either of our previously described podiums? It is not too tough a task to think of coaches as Platonic craftsmen, and competitors as raw materials to be shaped and constructed. At the risk of shining a light of undue superordinance on coaches, it is their sense of what an athlete *should be* that initiates and then guides the process leading to what that athlete *becomes*. Admittedly, very rarely do athletes knock on a coach's door and offer themselves as blank slates. However, even more rarely do coaches accept an athlete into their tutelage and bend their methodology to whatever the athlete wishes to do on some given day.[15] It seems fair, then, to consider the coach to be the cabinetmaker, and the athlete the fine-aged piece of cherry to be hand-sawn and chiseled into a competitive piece of furniture, or even a champion athlete.

When Socrates' blacksmith sets out to create a drill, he does so intending to create the perfect drill. So too does a coach intend to utilize his knowledge of a given sport to shape his athlete into that athlete's most perfect instantiation of that sport's athletic Form. It is only with some sense of a Form of what a perfect athlete is that a coach can begin construction of a physical copy. If a coach bases his process on an imperfect model, even if that imperfect model is the best athlete in the world in the same given sport, then his own athlete can only ever hope to achieve a similar status as an imperfect athlete.

To put this point more philosophically, as The Allegory of the Cave teaches, to focus on and model a coaching method on the results of a client competitor is to be practicing imperfection. If a coach formulates a series of methods meant to produce in his athletes some result that focuses only on besting some fellow-competitor, then the pinnacle of achievement would be edging out that fellow-competitor; an achievement that would rely too much on a plethora of uncontrollable issues. Assuming similar methods, which is the most likely result when focusing on imitating a fellow-competitor, which in turn is the most likely result when making one's goal *to beat the fellow-competitor*, the natural set of talents of each athlete becomes the controlling factor in the competition. Thus, uncontrollable issues such as wind-speed (in some race); or randomized bracket placement (in some tournament); or flip of a coin (in deciding possession order) can be the deciding factor in that competition.

For example, there have been numerous instances in which a weightlifter who was not even competing in the A group (or top seeded tier) earned a gold, silver, or bronze medal, despite not posting qualifying lifts to earn them the opportunity to compete on the premier stage.[16] If that B or C group lifter was focused only on the competitor to his left or right then that lifter would probably not even come close to hitting the A group numbers required to win a medal.

However, if a coach takes Plato's advice, and makes his goal the *perfection* of the *athlete*, regardless of what he may believe it takes just to beat some other athlete, then the relative importance of the uncontrollable issues diminishes because the coach's athlete has a more substantial set of methods on which to draw. It is only those who are still dwelling in Plato's cave that focus on what others are doing. Once out of the cave and into the light, a coach and his athlete can focus on exactly what it is that takes one from functioning as a competitor that focuses on and adjusts her training to that of a similarly imperfect competitor to one who models herself after a more perfect Form of an Ideal Competitor.

If a competitor focuses her efforts on attaining the sort of perfection present in the realm of the Forms, she may end up more perfect than the competitor who focuses her efforts on becoming nothing more than the best of her fellow competitors: those imperfect shadows on the competition cave's wall. But if she sets out intending only to be better than some imperfect shadow on the cave wall, attaining the sort of perfection found in the realm of the Forms is not even a possibility. Thus, the best that she can hope for is something out of her control to be the deciding factor in that competition. And, as we have determined, minimizing the uncontrollable is just as crucial to success as maximizing the controllable. And there is no athlete or coach in the world, regardless of sport or level of competition, who prefers less control over any aspect of training, competition preparation, or competition itself. By striving to stand atop the podium on which the lower platforms are inhabited by inferior versions of oneself, the athlete maximizes her control over her chances to stand atop the podium inhabited by other athletes as well.

On Avoiding Sun and Sea: Ovid's Warning to Remain Dispassionate

> *Now Delos, Paros on the left are seen,*
> *And Samos, favour'd by Jove's haughty queen;*
> *Upon the right, the isle Lebynthos nam'd,*
> *And fair Calymne for its honey fam'd.*
> *When now the boy, whose childish thoughts aspire*
> *To loftier aims, and make him ramble high'r,*
> *Grown wild, and wanton, more embolden'd flies*
> *Far from his guide, and soars among the skies.*
> *The soft'ning wax, that felt a nearer sun,*
> *Dissolv'd apace, and soon began to run.*
> *The youth in vain his melting pinions shakes,*
> *His feathers gone, no longer air he takes:*
> *Oh! Father, father, as he strove to cry,*
> *Down to the sea he tumbled from on high,*
> *And found his Fate; yet still subsists by fame,*
> *Among those waters that retain his name.*[17]

In one of the fullest treatments of the fabled Icarus, Ovid—in his *Metamorphoses*—tells the tale of the son of Daedalus failing to heed his father's instruction to "take care To wing your course along the middle air; If low, the surges wet your flagging plumes; If high, the sun the melting wax consumes."

Instead, Daedalus advises Icarus, "Steer between both: nor to the northern skies, Nor south Orion turn your giddy eyes; But follow me: let me before you lay Rules for the flight, and mark the pathless way."

As we know, Icarus, overtaken by his childish thoughts, flew too close to the sun before falling into the sea, drowning after his wax wings melted. This tale perhaps too obviously reflects the danger Icarus faced when he flew too high to the detriment of the cautionary flipside of flying too low where the sea's surges would dampen the plumage and pull the boy into the water. Daedalus carefully warned his son of the equal perils of flying too high and too low. If Ovid would have crafted his tale slightly differently, the lesson learned would not have been one of avoiding hubris, but one of fending off discouragement, despondency, or some other similar interpretation of the hazard one faces when not keeping oneself up in order to avoid the jealous grasp of the depths of the hungry sea.

Written over a millennium earlier, Plato's *Cratylus* is a dramatic dialogue featuring its namesake, Cratylus, his philosophical opponent Hermogenes, and Plato's featured mouthpiece, Socrates. The three philosophers spend the work debating the various merits and drawbacks of naming conventions, specifically whether words for things are based on conventional agreements or a thing's natural usage. According to Hermongenes "whatever anyone decides to call a particular thing is its name."[18] For Cratylus, "things have natural names."[19] Socrates by the end appears to fall somewhere in the middle saying "both convention and usage must contribute something to expressing what we mean when we speak."[20] Socrates elaborates that he prefers the view "that names should be as much like things as possible" but that he fears "that defending this view is like hauling a ship up a sticky ramp...and that we have to make use of this worthless thing, convention, in the correctness of names."[21]

Socrates spends a good portion of *Cratylus* dispelling Hermogenes of the notion that there is no correct name for a thing other than what each man calls that thing, from community to community or country to country.[22] One method Socrates uses is getting Hermogenes to acknowledge that, irrespective of what a thing might be called, that thing has some "fixed being or essence" of its own.[23] While it does matter what words we use to refer to a thing, it only matters when we are trying to communicate some inquiry or proposition about that thing. The thing itself does not have the capacity to concern itself with what it is called. Rather, the fixed essence or being of things bears no "relation to us and are not made to fluctuate by how they appear to us. They are by themselves, in relation to their own being or essence, which is theirs by nature."[24]

To prove his theory of language, Socrates asks Hermogenes to consider various tools used in different activities.

> *Suppose, for example, that we undertake to cut something. If we make the cut in whatever way we choose and with whatever tool we choose, we will not succeed in cutting. But in each case we choose to cut in accord with the nature of cutting and being cut and with the natural tool for cutting, we'll succeed and cut correctly. If we try to cut contrary to nature, however, we'll be in error and accomplish nothing.*[25]

Similarly, Socrates goes on, "if we undertake to burn something, our burning mustn't accord with every belief but with the correct one—that is to say, with the one that tells us how that thing burns and is burned naturally, and what the natural tool for burning is."[26]

The underlying theme of Plato's *Cratylus* is the correctness of names, but in carving closer and closer to the name bone, Socrates teaches us another important lesson: the importance of dispassionate usage of tools. As Ovid cautions in "The Story of Daedalus and Icarus" following one's passion at the cost of the correct application of one's tools (in Icarus's case through hubris) tends to result in folly. Icarus failed to heed his father's warning that flying either too high or too low will require something of the boy's waxen wings that those wings were not designed to provide. It did not matter that Icarus wanted his wings to support his journey to advised-against altitudes; not even Daedalus's craftsmanship could design a wax that would withstand the sun's heat. It may have been the case that Icarus got so wrapped up in his flight that he forgot about his father's warnings, or it may have been the case that the boy remembered but cared more about flying higher than he did about the limits of his tools. Ovid only tells us that Icarus's "childish thoughts aspire(d) to loftier aims and (made) him ramble high'r" until he grew "wild, and wanton," stressing his wings beyond their tolerance.

A similar theme develops when Socrates is helping Hermogenes along to the point of agreeing that a thing's proper use does not depend on what we want from it. Icarus does not get to use his wings to fly to the sun just like a craftsman "mustn't make the tool in whatever way he happens to choose, but in the natural way."[27] More reasonable is the craftsman who, when he "discovers the type of tool that is naturally suited for a given type of work" embodies that tool "in the material out of which he is making the tool."[28] In this way Socrates' craftsman starts with an end goal and chooses his tool based on the goal he is trying to attain. The craftsman does not look around at his tools and decide to use them in a way that he sees fit if that method is incongruent with the craftsman's desired outcome.

Just as a thing's fixed essence or being does not depend on what we feel about it or want from it, neither does the effectiveness of our tools depend on how we feel about them or want from them. Our comfort with a tool—perhaps in our case a barbell, a dumbbell, or a particular movement or set or rep scheme—is not what guarantees the effective or ineffective accomplishment of our training mission. One athlete may find a groove in which she performs high weight, low repetition snatches four days per week, high weight, low repetition clean and jerks four days per week, and low weight, high repetition back squats six days per week with little assistance work in the meantime. Another athlete may feel more comfortable with some variation on that theme in which she substitutes low weight, high repetition back squats with moderate weight, low repetition front squats. And all of these athletes will enjoy varying degrees of success, none of which is necessarily *inherently* tied to the comfort level of each athlete. Rather, the degrees of success will depend on the effectiveness of the programming and the intensity of and degree of skill with which each movement is performed. The point of this analysis is not to evaluate the various merits of programming strategies but to help diagnose potential problems in becoming too passionate about one or another way of approaching success given the tools we are familiar with.

Crucially, we must not focus our attention only on theoretical tools like programming or training modalities; a similar predicament may more obviously manifest itself in overreliance on certain physical tools. At the end of a training cycle—assuming competition is the end-state of that cycle—a maximum weight single snatch and maximum weight single clean and jerk are the only movements a weightlifter cares about and needs to focus his energies on. But how he arrives at a peak performance on the competition platform may require a dramatically more varied or narrowed focus relative to what he prefers or is comfortable with.

There is only so much one can expect from focusing on a specific movement such as a front squat. There is only so much one can hope to get out of maxing out every movement five days a week. And—despite everything a purist might hold fast to—a barbell will only improve a weightlifter's total so much. To be as clear as possible, this is not a rallying cry to replace snatch pulls with sit-ups or barbells with stationary bikes. On the contrary, there are likely many athletes and laylifters who should be focusing more on classic movements like high weight, low repetition snatches, clean and jerks, and front and back squats. Just as old-school devotees may be passionate to the point of overreliance on these schemes and movements, so too might one wish to avoid the discomfort that accompanies the fundamental movements in favor of accessory work that focuses on piecemealing the classic lifts together in a more agreeably comfortable fashion.

Regardless of whether a weightlifter prefers the historical programming and movements or some variation on nouveau accessory theories, each should learn from Ovid and Socrates that any tools we might have available to us do not care what we expect from them. Because at the end of each training day, that is all a program or a barbell is, a tool; a tool that does not respond to our hubris or complacency. And when the tool utilized ceases to produce some desired result, then it may be time to reconsider whether that tool's fixed being or essence is able to provide what we need from it or whether it is time to change our feathers in order to avoid the sun and sea and instead wing our course along the middle air.

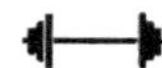

On Embracing Stoicism Through Injury and Triumph

In 1999 Greg Calhoon and Andrew C. Fry analyzed six years of data sets of reported injuries suffered by athletes in various sports at the Olympic Training Centers. The data showed that the injuries suffered by male weightlifters were primarily overuse injuries, rather than traumatic injuries that affected joint integrity. Calhoon and Fry determined that both the "injury patterns and rates were similar to those reported for other sports and activities."[29] The majority of the injuries reported were to the lower back, knees, and shoulders and—fortunately for the athletes and their careers— "the recommended number of training days missed for most injuries was 1 day or fewer."[30] The athletes studied reported injuries at a rate of 3.3 injuries per 1,000 hours of weightlifting. However, it may be the case that the competitive performance of sport specific movements results in higher rates of injury than what Calhoon and Fry uncovered in their study of weightlifting training.

A decade after Calhoon and Fry's paper another group of authors published a paper analyzing "the frequency, characteristics, and causes of injuries incurred during the Summer Olympic Games" in Beijing in 2008. In the Olympic study 88% of the nearly 11,000 registered Olympians reported 1,055 injuries; "an incidence of 96.1 injuries per 1,000 registered athletes." There, 72.5% of the injuries were incurred in competition with nearly half of the injuries preventing the athlete from further competition or training. Unlike the training study, the Olympic study found that only 22% of reported injuries resulted from overuse, while one-third were caused by contact with another athlete. Interestingly, weightlifting was the only solo, non-contact sport listed among the sports with the highest risk of injury; the others being soccer, taekwondo, hockey, handball, and boxing.[31]

None of this is likely very surprising to any weightlifter—competitive or otherwise—who has spent more than a few moments in either a training or competition environment. That the above studies found injury rates in weightlifting relatively similar to injury rates in other sports but more prevalent in the highest levels of competition is also rather intuitive: the higher the stakes, the more likely the injury.[32]

On the flip side of injury is the success and glory that comes with made lifts, podium appearances, and medals. At the highest level, one gold, one silver, and one bronze are awarded to the most successful athletes in their sport's competition and that only occurs once every four years (notwithstanding a strike, global pandemic, or world war). At the 2020 Summer Olympics in Tokyo, 42 individual athletes out of 197 were awarded a medal. In the 2019 World Weightlifting Championships in Pattaya, Thailand 588 athletes from 97 nations competed with 60 of those athletes earning a medal.[33] This means that, between the Olympics and the World Championships, roughly 13% of the participating athletes stood on a podium after all the weights were lifted and lowered.

What of the 87% of the participating athletes who did not medal on the world's biggest stages? Of that other 87% there may have been numerous competitors who lifted more weight than they had ever lifted before who simply had no chance to place in the top three in their weight classes simply based on the composition of each class. And what about the countless others who did not qualify for either the World Championships or the Olympics? They may have won other competitions like any of the numerous continental, national, regional, or local events found around the world. Or they may never have even registered to compete in any sanctioned events but find themselves making and missing lifts that both frustrate and gratify them in their own garage or basement just the same.

It might be tempting to wholly throw oneself into the glory of victories, but with such revelry comes the emotive tendency to wallow in the disgust or self-pity that comes with the inevitable defeats. To guard against these tendencies, it is not enough to be aware of the fact that emotion drives the train that carries both our highs and our lows; we also must recognize that we can learn to control that train and use its power in our favor, so long as we understand the switches that control the tracks on which both the glory and victory trains run.

There are some switches our minds are able to flip that will help us arrive at short term success while others are more useful for longer-term journeys. We can come quickly to know and understand the value of an even temper and steady resolve but the actualization and realization of either do not come immediately along with the recognition of their value. In Arrian's *Discourses of Epictetus*, Chapter XV asks us "if the fig tree's fruit is not brought to perfection suddenly in a single hour, would you gather fruit of men's minds so soon and so easily?" If the fruit is not easily or quickly bore, is it still worth harvesting? Epictetus seems to think so.

Earlier, in Book I Chapter I, Epictetus lays out his fundamental thesis that reason is the lone faculty we have received that was created to comprehend its own nature. Music, he says, will tell you about tunes, but it will not tell you whether you should or should not sing or play at any given moment. Grammar will tell you what words to write and in what arrangement but not whether you should or should not write to your friend. Reason is apart from music, grammar, or any other faculty because reason says "what it is and what it can do, and with what precious qualities it has come to us, and to comprehend all other faculties as well."[34] Where the music tells us a song is arranged well and grammar whether a sentence is coherent, reason is what tells us we should sing if we like and write if we wish.

31

This reason and our ability to use it is the central distinction between man and animal. The gods gave us reason to master our other faculties, unlike animals which are slaves to their passions. Man has his body in common with animals, and reason and intelligence in common with the gods.[35] In this way man's ability to reason puts him in touch with the gods and, as such, using reason to master passion makes man more godlike than animal like.

Never too far from another of our faculties—our memories—are the missed PRs, questionable red lights, and disastrous physical setbacks that have impeded our progress or the progress of our partners or friends. Likely right beside those memories are the flashes of anger, despair, or depression that accompanied each unhappy moment or series of moments. Remember that for those who compete in some professional-ish capacity—therefore exhibiting an expected level of expertise the laylifter likely does not hold—3.3 injuries occur for every 1,000 hours of training, mostly due to overuse (with that frequency and severity go up at the higher levels). While emotions like anger, despair, or depression are perfectly reasonable reactions to both misses and injury, Epictetus teaches us that giving into such passions makes us like an animal that cannot evaluate its actions because none of the results happened within our *will*. But crucially, the same is true for the elation we feel and see in others when big lifts are made, PRs are hit, and medals are placed around the necks of those on podiums. Remember also that only 13% of the participants in the World Weightlifting Championships and Olympic win medals, and that there are countless millions of others who never even come close to experiencing the joy that comes with both reaching and succeeding at such paramount levels. As saddening as it may be to put down on paper or say out loud, success in Olympic weightlifting is far more fleeting than failure. Therefore, it is just as important to guard ourselves against giving into the emotions that attend success as it is to insulate ourselves from those that come with failure.

Only when we follow the Stoics who show us that reason can guide us to the land of the gods who use that tool to master passion will we be able to center ourselves in a way that permits us to thrive in spite of our defeats and in caution against our successes. Epictetus reminds us that the fruits of thriving will not be reaped easily, but they will be worth harvesting. Reason alone will not be what we lean on to guard ourselves against the danger of high and low reactions to victory and defeat, but it will help us comprehend the importance of doing so. It will, in the end, be up to us to train our minds to operate as sharply as our hip hinges, third pulls, and foot positioning. There is no partitioning the mind and body in this regard; neither can work without the other. To pretend otherwise would be to live like an animal. To embrace this as truth is to lift among the gods.

On Selecting a Coach: The Systemic Art of Identifying the Sophist

Socrates: So, in a word, whenever a man considers a thing for the sake of another thing, he is taking counsel about that thing for the sake of which he was considering, and not about what he was investigating for the sake of something else.

Nicias: Necessarily so.

Socrates: Then the question we ought to ask with respect to the man who gives us advice, is whether he is expert in the care of that thing for the sake of which we are considering when we consider.

Nicias: Yes.

Socrates: Then the question whether any one of us is expert in the care of the soul and is capable of caring for it well, and has had good teachers, is the one we ought to investigate.

Laches: What's that, Socrates? Haven't you ever noticed that in some matters people become more expert without teachers than with them?

Socrates: Yes, I have, Laches, but you would not want to trust them when they said they were good craftsmen unless they should have some well-

*executed product of their art to show you—and
not just one but more than one.*[36]

Outside of the vanishingly small number of professional athletes whose livelihoods rely on their competitive performances, the remaining majority of laylifters enjoys a greater margin of error around their learning and movements. For example, there are not enough lifetimes for a professional weightlifter to master both a left leg forward and right leg forward split jerk. There is typically a more natural forward leg for every weightlifter, whether lay or professional, but actual mastery of both methods would take more time, effort, and refinement than any one individual has time to devote. The same must also be said for holistic approaches to the movements involved in the sport itself.

For most athletes across the entire skill set spectrum technical progress will best be realized by hiring some sort of instructor. To transform herself from a novice lifter to an intermediate lifter she must learn a set of skills that an intermediate lifter will not have to doubly learn in order to transition from intermediate to advanced. Basic footwork and eyeline and hip placement should be mastered before more technical proficiencies such as elbow rotation and weight distribution. Similarly, these latter movements will most likely be realized prior to even more advanced concepts like barbell vacillation timing and variable torso angling throughout a jerk's dip and drive. Similarly, just as each lifter needs to learn, understand, and acquire some level of mastery over each foundation of a snatch and clean and jerk prior to seeking out the more advanced concepts, an instructor must be proficient not only in the understanding of the relevant concepts, but in the relative needs of each athlete.[37] To best understand how a lifter might best position himself to move from one phase of his career to the next under the proper instructor's guidance, we can use a method Plato offers in his book *Sophist* in which Socrates and his fellow philosophers distinguish between a teacher who is good for the soul and one who is, perhaps, merely "an expert at deception."[38]

In another of Plato's books, *Phaedrus*, Socrates refers to this method of inquiry as a "systemic art."[39] By first "seeing together things that are scattered about everywhere and collecting them into one kind" the philosopher is able to "make clear the subject of any instruction" he wishes to give.[40] Next, the inquiry permits us to "cut up each kind according to its species along its natural joints" being careful "to try not to splinter any part."[41] Socrates himself uses this method of inquiry in his treatment of pleasure and knowledge in one of Plato's last books, *Philebus*. In *Philebus* Socrates is careful to warn Protarchus that opposites are sometimes part of the same thing. While "black is not only different from white but is in fact its very opposite," they are both colors.[42] And while shapes may "differ in innumerable ways," shapes are "all one in genus."[43]

We do not have to spend entire books applying this system of division and collection to weightlifters and their coaches in order to find out what Plato might say about the relationship between those two parties. But it is helpful to understand that, in order for an individual athlete to maximize the value of his relationship with a potential coach, and that not all coaches are equally fit to the needs of all athletes, there is certainly a specific category of teachers all types of athletes should learn to recognize in order to avoid.

We can begin building our Platonic system by collecting all weightlifters and lumping them into one group: those who seek to pick up a barbell up, put that barbell over their heads, and then put that barbell back down, in the form of a snatch and a clean and jerk. We can then divide that group into four categories: novice, intermediate, expert, and professional. Regardless of the category into which each of our group falls, we can hypothesize that, at some point in an athlete's career—irrespective of whether that athlete ever advances beyond the novice stage—that athlete will more probably than not benefit from some outside instruction.

Weightlifting coaches, likewise, can be lumped into one elemental group: those who seek to impart some instruction on another in order to, at least ostensibly, help that other improve her ability to perform the snatch and clean and jerk.

And the stage at which an athlete will most likely benefit from the broadest possible category of coaches is at the novice level. This is because no athlete is ever an intermediate, expert, or professional weightlifter without first paying her dues as a novice. Because all weightlifters are at some point novices, they are the most likely to benefit from outside instruction. This does not mean that the benefit an expert derives from outside instruction is not more valuable than the instruction a novice derives. This only suggests that the stage at which we find the group most likely to benefit is with the novices.

Simplistically speaking we can further divide novice lifters into four groups:

1. those who choose to go it alone and figure out the movements without either lay assistance or professional instruction and forever forge their own athletic paths
2. those who begin their lifting tenures as a 1 before moving onto a 3
3. those who seek either lay assistance or professional instruction to learn the basics and then take their lifting lives into their own hands for good
4. those who seek either lay assistance to learn the basics before subsequently obtaining professional instruction to further master the movements or begin with professional instruction and maintain that relationship for the duration of their lifting lives

This whole exercise may seem exhausting, just as it surely exhausted the Eleanic visitor with whom Socrates sought to determine precisely what a *sophist* is.[44] But the benefit of this system outweighs its mental toll because it offers exactly what it is we are after: a thorough accounting of what is and is not the type of coach that maximizes each weightlifter's individual athletic needs.

Regardless of the category into which either a novice or advanced athlete fits—either neatly or haphazardly—one of the enduring issues all athletes face is where to and to whom to turn for help. Due to a seemingly everlasting increase in the number of coaches and various other types of instructors the idea of selecting the optimal teacher can be quite overwhelming for one who may not have a fundamental understanding of what an instructor should bring to a coach-student relationship. Rather than focusing first on what one *should* look for in a teacher, we might first throw all possible instructors in an educational funnel and work to siphon out the undesirables by determining what we should *not* look for or—more accurately—how not to look for one.

With the advent of the Internet and its branches of supposed intelligentsia—message boards, social media, online certifications and so on—knowing where and to whom to turn for trustworthy instruction is dangerously overwhelming. As much as it is for the better that lifters in all four of our categories can find instructional articles, videos, and curated and personalized coaching in almost any preferred medium, it is equally for the worse that in each of those media those lifters can find some kernel of information that either confirms their preconceived notions of what the right answers to their questions might be as well as truly horrific advice or instruction dressed up like brilliant guidance. Most dangerous of all, though, is the material that appears well-reasoned, tried, tested, and true, but is nothing more than some less egregious version of the brilliantly packaged horror that passes as snake oil.

Quite often the hucksterism behind the message, even if appetizingly presented, can give itself away under some cursory scrutiny. If, for example, a coach promises she can add 5kg to any lifter's clean and jerk with just three simple tricks, not much scholastic inquiry is required to guess that there is something fantastic about her claim. There is simply no physical way that any coach, no matter how skilled or studied she is, can guarantee such progress to every lifter across all skillsets. Such incredible claims, though, are much easier to discern than those made by teachers who advertise no concrete guarantees but still offer fundamentally groundless instruction that serves a student no better than the more obviously ridiculous 5kg-for-all promise.

Such false prophets can be found in all fields of instruction but, when it comes to an activity like weightlifting—one with so many variables that even the most coherent and credentialed coaches cannot guarantee success—

determining which teachers are worthy of followers and which should be ignored is particularly distressing.[45] When there is no guaranteed physically measurable or tangible metric for the validity of a proposition we are left to reason our way to the truth or falsity of an idea. Prior to the formalizing of systematic analyses of logic, those skilled in rhetoric—specifically utilizing rhetoric to convey false teachings—were called *sophists*.[46]

In his inquiry into what precisely a sophist is, Plato recounts a meeting between Socrates, Theatetus, and a visiting philosopher from the Greek town of Elea.[47] In *Sophist* Theatetus and the visitor spend the beginning of their conversation differentiating between that which is not from that which is but is not the genuine form of the thing sought. One may not be a coach at all, and another may be a coach but is not the form of a coach an athlete is seeking:

> *Theaetetus: What in the world would we say a copy is, sir, except something that's made similar to a true thing and is another thing that's like it?*
> *Visitor: You're saying it's another true thing like it? Or what do you mean by like it?*
> *Theaetetus: Not that it's true at all, but that it resembles the true thing.*
> *Visitor: Meaning by true, really being?*
> *Theaetetus: Yes.*
> *Visitor: And meaning by not true, contrary of true?*
> *Theaetetus: Of course.*
> *Visitor: So you're saying that that which is like is not really that which is, if you speak of it as not true.*
> *Theaetetus: But it is, in a way.*
> *Visitor: But not truly, as you say.*
> *Theaetetus: No, except that it really is a likeness.*

> *Visitor. Maybe that which is not is woven together with that which is in some way like that—it's quite bizarre.*[48]

Theaetetus immediately agrees with the visitor's estimation that the sophist is an expert at deception because the sophist "makes our souls believe what is false."[49] The important thing to note here is not that the sophist is not an expert. It would be far easier for a student to identify those teachers not worth listening to if such teachers were simply unskilled or amateurish. Unfortunately, according to Plato, the sophist is such a proficient teacher that his ability to impress the object of his teaching upon his subject renders him just as much of an expert as the teacher who passes along truths and goodness.

This expertise exhibited by the sophist demonstrates his seemingly endless supply of confusing objections to false teachings. Whereas the visitor is engaging Theaetetus in Theaetetus's own education by means of this systemic art of division and collection, the expert teacher of falsities offers his students something like the truth but is not really the truth at all. The visitor, rather, refuses to permit Theaetetus to accept, without deeper investigation, whatever definitions the visitor offers for what a sophist is and does. The visitor explicitly acknowledges the difficulty inherent in this sort of mode of education. He openly worries that Theaetetus will find the visitor insane for repeatedly taking one position then another for the sake of refuting that which is untrue.[50] In his condensed history *The Story of Philosophy*, Will Durant agrees that "Some who suffered from this 'Socratic Method,' this demand for accurate definitions, and clear thinking, and exact analysis, objected that he asked more than he answered, and left men's minds more confused than before."[51] But while this is a worrisome feature of what has become known as the Socratic method of instruction, it is certainly just that: a feature.[52]

The key difference between the sophist and the Socratic, both of whom may tend to confuse their pupils, is that the sophist does it to obfuscate the truth about his instruction: that it leads to deception, not truth. This

Socratic method, while perhaps similarly confusing, is utilized to help bring a student closer to the truth by identifying and evaluating as many propositions as possible in order to determine that which is most virtuous.

Whether we are reading Plato telling us the story of Socrates, Theaetetus, and their visitor working together to identify the wicked properties of sophists as teachers of deception or working to determine for ourselves to whom we should turn for that ever elusive missing link between our second and third pull, one truth is constant: the good and virtuous teacher will constantly try to get us to the truth while the sophist will strive to corrupt the pathway to truth by mapping our reality onto that which is false no differently than the way the deceitful coaches confuse their clients and lead them away from proper movement instruction.

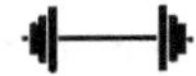

On The Ship of Theseus: Ourselves v. Ourselves

[For, according to Heraclitus, it is not possible to step twice into the same river, nor is it possible to touch a mortal substance twice in so far as its state is concerned. But, thanks to the swiftness and speed of change,] it scatters <things> and brings <them> together again, [(or, rather, it brings together and lets go neither again nor later, but simultaneously)] it forms and dissolves, and it approaches and departs.[53]

This fragment from the pre-Socratic Greek philosopher, Heraclitus, laid the philosophical foundation for one of the longest standing and most recognizable thought experiments in all of metaphysics, The Ship of Theseus. Before the Greek philosopher and father of biography, Plutarch, popularized Heraclitus's idea of the ebb and flow of identity, Socrates, in Plato's *Cratylus*, referred to the fragment when discussing the nature of naming conventions with Hermogenes, pointing out that "those who use the name *ōsia*[54] seem to agree pretty much with Heraclitus' doctrine that the things that are all flowing and that nothing stands fast—for the cause and originator of them is then the pusher and so is well named *ōsia*."[55]

Plutarch, born nearly five centuries after Plato, allegorized the identity puzzle in his biography of Theseus, King of Athens:

> *"The ship wherein Theseus and the youth of Athens returned had thirty oars, and was preserved by the Athenians down even to the time of Demetrius Phalereus, for they took away the old planks as they decayed, putting in new and stronger timber in their place, insomuch that this ship became a standing example among the philosophers, for the logical question of things that grow; one side holding that the ship remained the same, and the other contending that it was not the same."*[56]

If scholarly estimates are correct that Demetrius Phalereus was born around 350 BC, then Theseus's ship would have stood for roughly nine centuries.[57] Irrespective of lifespans of various ancient Greek timber species, the only way that sort of longevity is possible is through careful repair and replacement of rotting or otherwise corrupted planks, as Plutarch describes. The philosophical puzzle, he offers, is whether the ship, after all of the original planks had eventually been replaced, is still the Ship of Theseus.

It takes no dramatic intellectual compromise to agree that if one or two planks out of a couple hundred are replaced, the ship is still substantially the same ship as it was before the one or two planks were replaced. Over time, as more of the original planks are replaced, the ship begins to lose its original identity and is less obviously the same ship; whatever definition of *same* one might hold. Finally, as every plank has been replaced, we fully realize Plutarch's puzzle: is the ship still the same ship, is it an entirely new ship, or is it some hybrid version of original and replacement?[58]

The identity puzzle is mind-bending enough when we are discussing mythical Greek ships but how about when we ask the same questions of ourselves? Are our corporal bodies the same bodies as they were when we were younger? If so, would our bodies be the same if enough of our organs were replaced through medical transplants? Or we dyed our hair or lost a limb? If not, at what age did our current bodies become distinctly different from our younger bodies? Was it a marked occasion like the loss of a tooth? Or was every fraction of an inch that we grew sufficient to render our new height characteristic of a new version of ourselves?

Unlike Heraclitus, who contends that no man can step in the same river twice, Plutarch does not offer an answer to his puzzle. But what he does give us is even better: a tool for introspection that allows us not only to ask whether the *we* of today is the same as the *we* of yesterday, last week, or last year. We are also able to remind ourselves that there is no static version of ourselves against which to measure progress made or lost on a day-to-day scale.

The first day any of us stepped into a fitness facility of any sort was likely the same as it was for everyone else: confusing, intimidating, or at least overwhelming. The resolve it took for us to look at the behemoths on the platforms hoisting uncountable kilograms of molded rubber in the air and say *I can do that too* should never be discounted. Going again back to whatever our motives might have been, whether we wanted to learn the snatch and clean and jerk from the ground up, use those movements to better our overall athletic performance, or to put finer points on an already competitive skill set acquired at home or in a different gym, it is almost certainly unlikely that we are today the same lifters we were when we decided to surround ourselves with other, better weightlifters and coaches.

For most proficient lifters, keeping track of day-to-day or season-to-season progress is second nature; a habit that may not have come naturally or intuitively but one we can no longer imagine living without. Somewhere scratched in those weeks or months or years of logbooks we can see the construction, destruction, and reconstruction of the Ships of Us. The day one you is not the day now you but there has never been a day where you were not you. Throughout the entirety of one's weightlifting tenure the movements have been learned and pieced together. Those pieced-together movements have been sanded down in order that the pieces fit more seamlessly together than their original haphazard positioning that was the likely natural outcome of simply watching another lifter move a barbell from the ground, place it in a hip pocket, and then pull it overhead before awkwardly attempting to recreate the same flow ourselves. Only after struggling through session after session is one able to more coherently orient the various pulls and pushes comprising highly technical weightlifting movements. But what would Plutarch say about you as a weightlifter? Or, more importantly, what would Plutarch's take on the Ship of Theseus help us understand about ourselves as weightlifters?

We find a useful hint in yet another version of this puzzle in Plato's *Parmenides* in which Plutarch's fellow Greek offers a slightly different take on the task:

> *"But if the one and the same were identical, whenever anything became the same it would always become one, and when it became one, the same." "Certainly." "Then if the one is the same with itself, it will not be one with itself; and thus, being one, it will not be one; this, however, is impossible; it is therefore impossible for one to be either the other of other or the same with itself."..."Impossible." "Thus the one cannot be either other or the same to itself or another." "No, it cannot." "And again it will not be like or unlike anything, either itself or another." "Why not?" "Because the like is that which is affected in the same way." "Yes." "But we saw that the same was of a nature distinct from that of the one."*[59]

Here Plato seems to take issue with whether the nature of a thing can be affected in the same way as the nature of a thing *like* it. In plainer words, does destroying or improving upon the Ship with newer and stronger timbers similarly destroy or improve upon the Ship with old, decaying planks? In our case we can imagine the answer being, anticlimactically, both yes and no.

For example, adding two kilos to a lifter's current 250kg total does not affect the nature of that lifter's total in the same way that adding two kilos did when that lifter's total was 100kg. For one thing, from what we understand of novice gains and linear progressions, strength improvements are more dramatic and easier to come by when a lifter's total is relatively low. Adding two kilos to the 100kg total is easier to do than adding the same absolute amount to the 250kg total, despite two kilos representing 2% of the lower total and 0.008% of the higher total. The same can be said about technical proficiencies. Improving upon one's bar path off the floor is crucial to second pull proficiency but much easier to come by than mastering the timing of front rack oscillation in a jerk. The bar path, however, is again representatively more dramatic than the oscillation mastery in that the efficiency of that portion of the lift must be learned before rack oscillation even comes into play. It is only once the bar moves up from the ground to the rack smoothly that the bar's movement up and down while in the rack even matters.

In each case, adding two kilograms to a total and sanding off the frictional edges to make a barbell flow more smoothly around a weightlifter's center of gravity affect both the first day novice and the current day athlete. Similarly we cannot say that the lifters we *were* are the same as or separate from the lifters we *are*. But understanding Heraclitus, Plutarch, and Plato can help us understand the path we and our barbells take and that, when we are evaluating ourselves as athletes, we must identify whether we are judging ourselves of today or the ourselves of our first day. Realistically, the ancient philosophers might say, there is a time and a place for each mode of introspection.

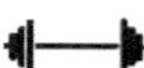

On Zeno and Aristotle: Every Lift is the Only Lift

Unlike Heraclitus' theory that everything is in a constant state of change[60] Parmenides proposes that being as a whole is continuous and that nothing that exists ever changes.[61] In contrast to the earlier idea that a man cannot step in the same river twice because of the river's swiftness and speed of change, Parmenides suggests that everything that exists is continuous, "motionless within the limits of great bonds."[62] So where Heraclitus might argue that a baby turns into a boy turns into a man, Parmenides may respond that from infancy to old age, the person is the person and size, shape, or muscular build differences do not change who that person was and is. Where we see a tree grow from a seed and wither into fertilizer, nothing in that process really comes into or goes out of existence; there is no process within the limits or boundaries of nature that we can refer to as change.

Parmenides is credited with founding the Eleatic School, a pre-Socratic school of philosophy that valued a logical construction of truth over a truth discovered by sensory experiences. Relying on a sensory experience of the world, our eyes see grass and trees growing and our hands feel the bark and leaves and soil, and we interpret that sensory input as a change in the landscape. The Eleatics, alternatively, viewed a sensory construction of truth as deceptive. Perhaps the grass and trees we are seeing are constructed copies made to look real and perhaps the bark and leaves and soil we feel are imitations made by artisans. For Parmenides and the Eleatics, we cannot always trust our eyes, but we can always trust reason. Because our senses sometimes fail us where logic does not, it is naive to believe that the world around us can be understood in any terms other than what our logical faculties prove.

The most famous student in the Eleatic School was Zeno of Elea, famous for his eponymous paradoxes. It is hard to overstate the role Zeno plays in the history of philosophy. In addition to the paradoxes Zeno manufactured, it is equally important to understand the manner in which Zeno wrote and the reason he produced the famous paradoxes that bear his name. Zeno was probably born around 490 BC. Beyond that we do not have a lot of information about his life outside of what Plato tells us in *Parmenides*, a dialogue featuring Socrates, Zeno, and Parmenides.[63] Socrates says that Zeno's writings are the same as Parmenides' but Zeno changes his arguments around "to fool us into thinking he is saying something different."[64] Zeno does acknowledge that his writing "comes to the defense of Parmenides' argument against those who try to make fun of it by claiming that, if it is one, many absurdities and self-contradictions result from that argument."[65] That *one* Zeno refers to is Parmenides' above stated assertion that being as a whole is a continuous, unchanging oneness.[66]

Rather than simply mount a standard defense of Parmenides' philosophy Zeno rather creatively imagined circumstances in which motion itself was impossible. By doing so Zeno did not necessarily set out to show that all change is impossible. Instead, Zeno argued directly against arguments against Parmenides. If Zeno can show that it is impossible to move from one point to a different point, how can we seriously suggest that an infant can grow into a man or an acorn into a tree? To prove that motion—and therefore change—is impossible, Zeno effectively perfects a method of argument now called *reductio ad absurdum*. This method relies on the Eleatic School's strict adherence to logic and reasoning in favor of sensory input and intuition. Employing the *reductio ad absurdum* method, Zeno aimed to show that if we begin with an agreeable set of conditions and follow a logical chain of arguments to an absurd conclusion, the set of conditions must therefore be false. Some of Zeno's most famous paradoxes in which the *reductio* method is employed include the Arrow Paradox, the Dichotomy Paradox, and the race between Achilles and the Tortoise. Because none of Zeno's works are known to have survived, we rely on other philosophers' writings—in the case of these paradoxes of motion, Aristotle—in order to understand his philosophies, or at least his arguments against those who attacked Parmenides' ideas.

Aristotle, in Book VI of his *Physics*, tells us that Zeno "says that if everything when it occupies an equal space is at rest, and if that which is in locomotion is always occupying such a space at any moment, the flying arrow is therefore motionless."[67] According to Zeno's Arrow Paradox, in order for an arrow to fly, the arrow must move from one place to another. However, at any given moment in time, the arrow must occupy some point in space. At each moment the arrow is not moving because it is occupying a point in space and is therefore at rest. If the arrow is at rest, then it cannot be moving to the next point in space, nor has it just arrived from some previous point. Logically, for Zeno, the arrow must never be moving at all.

Even if we were to grant that the arrow moves from one point in space to the next, Zeno goes on to show us that "that which is in locomotion must arrive at the half-way stage before it arrives at the goal."[68] This paradox, commonly called the Dichotomy Paradox, requires any object in motion to travel an infinite series of shorter distances before arriving at the endpoint of its intended path. Before an arrow shot from a bow at point A can arrive at the target point B, it must first travel to the point ½ way between A and B, a point we can call $A^{1/2}$. Even if it were to escape the frozen point in time and space described in the Arrow Paradox, the arrow then needs to travel to the point halfway between $A^{1/2}$ and the next halfway point between $A^{1/2}$ and the target point B, perhaps called $A^{1/4}$. From there the arrow must get to $A^{1/8}$ and so on and so forth. The arrow may continue—again if we grant it the ability to escape that frozen point in time and space—to traverse a series of halfway distances between the bow and its target, but it can never logically reach the target because it will forever have to continue to reach its next halfway point.

Finally, as Aristotle relates Zeno's instruction, assuming the slowest runner has any sort of a head start in front of the quickest runner, in such a race "the quickest runner can never overtake the slowest, since the pursuer must first reach the point whence the pursued started, so that the slower must always hold a lead."[69] This paradox features a sort of culmination of the propositions set forth in the Dichotomy and Arrow Paradoxes: even granting the escape from the frozen point in time and space and granting the closure on a target point by some moving object, Zeno argues that, so long as there is some measure of a head start granted to a slower moving object, a faster moving object will never be able to catch, let alone overtake, that slower moving object. Demonstrative though it may be, rather than shifting imageries to Achilles and the Tortoise, we can remain with our arrows to demonstrate the impossibility of motion. If we imagine an arrow shot from a bow at 200 feet per second—again granting for the sake of these arguments that arrows can move at all and further granting that arrows can actually reach targets—that arrow will reach a target 2,000 feet away in ten seconds. If a second arrow is shot from a bow at 400 feet per second, that arrow will reach the target in five seconds, assuming both arrows are shot from the same starting point, toward the same target, from the same bow, with the same velocity. Mathematically, the second arrow, traveling twice as fast, should reach the target in half the time it takes the first arrow to reach the target. However, Zeno objects, if that slower arrow is fired from its bow even a fraction of a second before the second arrow, that second arrow can never even reach the first arrow, to say nothing of reaching the target before it.

In the time it takes the faster arrow to catch up to the slower arrow's starting point, that slower arrow will then have moved some other distance closer to their target. The faster arrow will then have to close that gap while again the slower arrow continues to move closer to the target, leaving the faster arrow with another gap to close. As Zeno points out, the slower arrow must always hold the lead because the faster arrow must always reach the point where the slower arrow started, then occupies, then later occupies, and so on and so forth.

Zeno's paradoxes are artfully crafted in ways that are easy to understand if we follow their logic yet frustratingly incomprehensible if we rely on our intuition. We know that motion is possible because we go about our day to day lives moving from one place to another as necessary or desired. We also know that arrows—assuming proper tools and mechanics are employed—must eventually reach their target because arrows do not simply stop moving midflight. And, finally, we know that an arrow fired at a rate of speed twice that of another arrow fired from the same point will quickly overtake the slower arrow—so long as the slower arrow was not fired so much earlier than the quicker arrow that capture is *physically*, that is not to say *logically* impossible—because we have experienced faster movers pass slower movers all the time. The Eleatics would respond to our experiential rebuttals by asking whether our senses have ever deceived us. Have we ever been wrong about what we saw or otherwise experienced? If we have, then our senses are faulty and cannot always be trusted. After all, if we cannot trust them one time, how can we know when to ever trust them? But is there anything faulty in Zeno's logic? If not, then we must admit that motion, and therefore change, is impossible.

Since Zeno postulated his famous paradoxes, contemporary and modern philosophers as well as mathematicians and physicists have sought to formulate satisfactory refutations of the ancient Eleatic's ideas on motion. Aristotle himself argued that flying arrows are not necessarily motionless because "time is not composed of indivisible moments any more than any other magnitude is composed of indivisibles."[70] More specifically, Aristotle argues,

> *"Zeno's argument makes a false assumption in asserting that it is impossible for a thing to pass over or severally to come in contact with infinite*

things in a finite time. For there are two senses in which length and time and generally anything continuous are called 'infinite': they are called so either in respect of divisibility or in respect of their extremities. So while a thing in a finite time cannot come in contact with things quantitatively infinite, it can come in contact with things infinite in respect of divisibility: for in this sense the time itself is also infinite: and so we find that the time is occupied by the passage over the infinite is not a finite but an infinite time, and the contact with the infinites is made by means of moments not finite but infinite in number.[71]

More plainly, if the distances between A and B are infinite, perhaps time is infinite. And if time is infinite, then there is no good reason to think the arrow would not reach the target eventually and that the faster arrow could at some point over infinite distances and infinite passages of time overtake the slower arrow. A more appreciable and relatable response features Diogenes Laertius, biographer of philosophers, upon hearing the suggestion that there is no such thing as motion, simply getting up and walking away.[72]

None of this to say we are particularly concerned with arrows or tortoises. But we are concerned with how we can measure progress, if it can even be made at all. Zeno provides us with some interesting views on how time and space can be measured. We can imagine time as a series of moments strung together but still independent of each other. At each individual point on the landscape of moments, where Zeno imagines his arrow to freeze on its way to a target, everything in the universe can be viewed like a space-time snapshot. In each snapshot we can view life and its trappings outside the experience of living it. Doing so lets us evaluate where we were or what we were doing objectively without sensory experience influencing those evaluations.

Ever the dutiful recordkeepers, most weightlifters tend to keep detailed logs of their session by session sets and reps. If we were to take the numbers that correspond to all of the snatches, the clean and jerks, the front and back squats, and all the other accessory lifts throughout a lifter's entire career, we might be able to produce a graph that looks something like this:

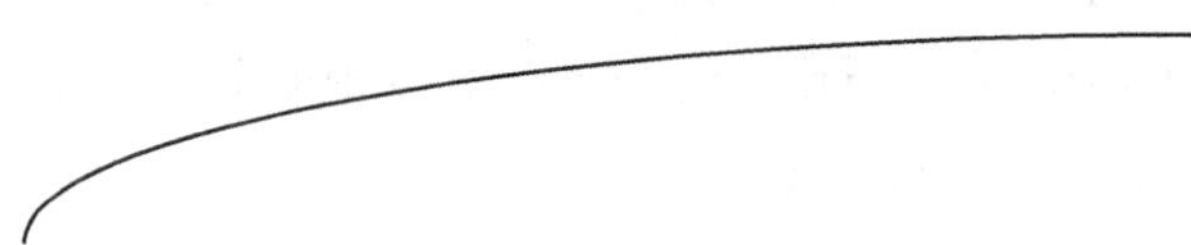

Over time our totals probably go up—at least at first and at least a little—relatively quickly. After these novice gains wear off and we begin to plateau we learn we need to alter our programming, technique, or both. Despite the fact that a few of our snatches and clean and jerks along the way might feel medal-worthy, for most of us the Olympic games are never a realistic objective. Sadly, no matter how hard we work, or for how long, we all—even the Olympians—hit a point where we simply cannot add any more weight to our lifts.

Broken down by year or season the logs of newer weightlifters produce results that track graphs showing an immediate upward trajectory before plateauing while later logs of more competitive lifters are more chaotic from session to session:

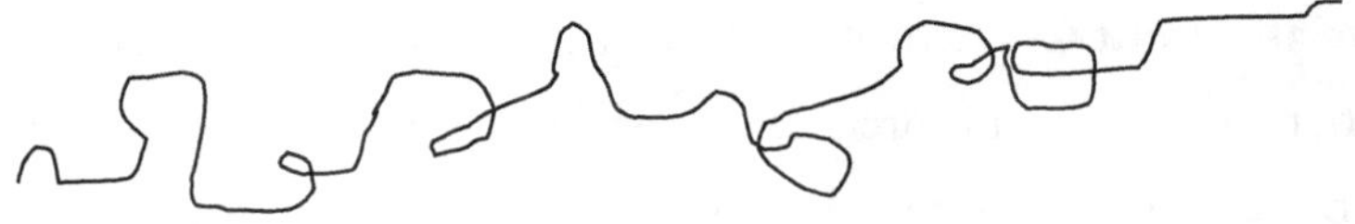

but ultimately higher rising than their novice counterparts. During competition, specifically, preparation typically involves pre-competition tapering that requires a weightlifter to lower the poundage on the barbell. And ideally, during competition itself, the athlete will hit the biggest numbers of her career, resulting in monumental spikes on her graph's landscape. Far more dramatic, however, for both laylifters and competitive weightlifters, are the individual sessions: those lifts Zeno teaches are frozen in time and space.

If we zoom in on our plot of sessions, we will see countless made snatches and missed clean and jerks and front squats that pinned us, and push presses not quite locked out. Every athlete knows the elation felt when a weight flies overhead that he has never lifted before. And, unfortunately, every athlete also knows the frustration of failing to set a new PR for longer than expected and, worse, the terror of worrying he may never PR again. But maybe we can learn something from Zeno that he did not necessarily intend to teach us.

If we visualize the larger arc of our lifetime of lifts as the path Zeno's Arrow takes on its way to its target, we can imagine each individual session as one of the moments in time and space that Zeno's Arrow occupies:

Breaking each individual session down even further into each attempt those dashes turn into dots that, when smashed back together to reframe a career's worth of snatch and clean and jerk attempts into a continuous arc, look just like our original figure. When we place our hands on the barbell and remind ourselves to keep our eyes up and wrap our fingers around our thumbs, the lift we are about to attempt effectively functions almost exactly as Zeno's Arrow: there was no lift before this one and there will be no lifts after. All that matters to us, all that exists in this place and at this time is this lift right here and right now. How we get to this point is not important, and neither is where we are going. Grasping the larger trajectory of our career's lifts up to such a point and beyond does not actually help us pick that barbell up and put it over our head. The entirety of our focus and all that matters is what is right in front of us. It can certainly be helpful in the moments surrounding each of our individual attempts to narrow our focus and forget all of the times we have failed at what we are about to do. It can even be helpful to forget about all of the times we have succeeded so that we do not become overconfident in our strength or complacent with our technique. Heeding Zeno's lessons and believing that there is no before or after and that progress is impossible allows us to treat every single lift like a gold medal depends on it. We will not get another chance because nothing will happen after this. But if we miss this lift, we can remind ourselves that, according to Zeno, such a lift never happened so there is no reason to doubt that we will make our next attempt at the same lift. However, as soon as we miss any attempt the fury and frustration work to return to suggest that we will never reach our target; the arrow fell out of the sky because motion is impossible.

But at that inevitable moment it is important to remind ourselves of Aristotle's response to Zeno—that if space is measured merely by a series of plot points on some continuum that makes motion and progress impossible then perhaps time itself occupies a similarly infinite series of points, allowing time and space to overlap, resulting in exactly the kind of progress Zeno's paradoxes prove are unthinkable. We must remember that the larger arc of thousands of lifts makes it easier for us to see that, over time, the individual missed attempts do not really hamper our lifetime of success. We see where we started, and we see where we finished, and we see that because we put in the requisite work we got stronger. Zeno's logical approach to the individual reps serves our mental preparation for the weight in front of us. And Aristotle's response aids our ability to overcome the individual failures by reminding us that, while that last lift may have been the only lift that existed, the next one will be too.

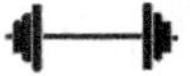

On Aesthetics: Plato and Pisarenko's Beautiful Lifts

An invariable difficulty when studying philosophy is working through texts that do not exactly translate to modern languages. Further difficulties arise when scholars debate to whom a work should even be attributed. One example of a work that typifies both of these hurdles is Plato's *Greater Hippias*, estimated to have been written sometime around 390 BC. While its authorship is still contested there is enough academic consensus that Plato probably did write *Greater Hippias* and that the work plays a central role in the development of a field of philosophy known as aesthetics.[73] The translation issue in *Greater Hippias* is additionally problematic but enjoys a greater consensus regarding the solution to how to adapt the ancient Greek *kalon* into modern language.

In *Greater Hippias* Socrates and a sophist called Hippias are discussing how to most appropriately evaluate parts of a speech; specifically, a speech Hippias gave that left Socrates unimpressed. The applicable term Hippias and Socrates are debating usage of, *kalos*, is popularly translated to the English word *fine*. While *fine* may seem a bit underwhelming to modern readers, the translation is variously described as "a widely applicable term of highly favorable evaluation covering our 'beautiful' (in physical, aesthetic, and moral senses), 'noble,' 'admirable,' 'excellent', and the like."[74] To avoid the rather uninspiring interpretation of the *fine* translation of *kalos* we will work through this discussion with the more popular—and accurate to the relevant philosophy—*beauty*. The dialogue in *Greater Hippias* features Socrates continually working to understand what attribute a thing, action, or person must have in order to be so highly valued that *kalos*, or *beautiful*, might apply.

Throughout Plato's works he identifies that which makes that which is beautiful beautiful as existing in the realm of Forms.[75] For Plato Beauty in its formal sense is eternal and absolute.[76] One attribute of Beauty itself, then, is its constancy; if Beauty exists then it is not subject to the sort of flux and change that actualized beautiful things are.[77] In *Greater Hippias* Socrates makes this distinction reminding Hippias that Hippias is not being asked what a beautiful thing is but what the Beautiful is. Hippias lamely responds that a beautiful girl is a beautiful thing.[78] Unsatisfied, Socrates asks Hippias to imagine the most beautiful mare, lyre, and pot and then to imagine the most beautiful of these next to the most beautiful girl and her next to the most beautiful of the gods. Hippias agrees then that, when compared to the gods, the human race is not beautiful.[79] Neither then does a beautiful pot compare to a beautiful girl, or a lyre to a pot or a mare to a lyre. Rather, the most beautiful in each category would appear foul compared to the most beautiful in the *more* beautiful category according to the hierarchy Socrates and Hippias build.

Hippias attempts to rebut Socrates' argument by forming a sophist's response that Beauty is the thing that, when added to a foul thing, makes it beautiful.[80] But Socrates, unsatisfied with Hippias's sophistry, wonders what we would say if we added something that made something in one category beautiful to something in different category. For instance, gold makes a statue more beautiful, but a golden spoon is not preferable to a spoon made of wood from a figtree.[81] No matter how beautiful gold might be, then, nor how effectively gold makes a statue more beautiful when gold is added to the statue, Beauty must not be the attribute Socrates is searching for because it does nothing to make a spoon more beautiful.

To clarify his query Socrates suggests three types of beauty: appropriateness[82], usefulness[83], and a specific type of usefulness that is in some way related to goodness.[84] Beauty must be appropriate because if what we conceive of as beautiful is misapplied, as in the case of a beautiful statute being used as a table, then we would really have neither a beautiful statute nor a beautiful table. Beauty must be useful because if a beautiful thing could not be used in some way, then the usable version of that same thing would definitionally be more beautiful than the thing that could not be used. And, finally, in order to be beautiful, that useful thing must be used for good. If we were to take a beautiful statue and use it to break a window, then the statue would not be realizing its potential beauty, at least as a statue.[85]

Beauty in the sense that Hippias and Socrates are investigating it differs from the perfect Beauty in the realm of Plato's Forms in that, in order for Socrates' usefulness criterion to be realized, the beautiful thing has to be not just an unrealized prototype but an instantiated form of a beautiful thing that we can enjoy. Like Hippias, it is easy to simply say that we can know Beauty by our experience with beautiful things. And, to some degree, Hippias is right. Describing attendance at an ancient Olympic event the Greek Stoic Epictetus said that even despite the imperfect "noise, clamor, and other disagreeable things" the "magnificence of the spectacle" made the games at ancient Olympia a work of God.[86] But imperfections such as noise and clamor, as well as pushy crowds and no comfortable places to bathe, are only permitted to correspond with beauty when appropriate. If we are participating in the ultimate physical competition, specifically the Olympics, we are willing to take the foulness that comes with imperfection and still be willing to call what we are seeing and hearing and feeling beautiful so long as it is appropriate. We would not be similarly willing to call an experience beautiful if it featured the same foulness—noisy, clamorous, and otherwise disagreeable—if what we were experiencing was not as beautiful as an experience like the one Epictetus describes at the Olympic games.

We find an additional perspective on appropriate Beauty when we consider the timing or placement of a beautiful movement. In weightlifting we can find examples of appropriate, useful, and good beauty in every garage and gym and on every platform; all beautiful without being perfect. Take Yurik Vardanyan's 182.5kg snatch at the 1984 Friendship Games in Varna, Bulgaria. With a first pull so smooth off the ground that his bottom position could have been held for however long it took to stabilize the world record weight overhead, the lift earned him the best snatch in the light heavyweight class. Soon after, we could hardly find fault in the nearly impeccable bar path and lockout of Vardanyan's 224kg clean and jerk. The shaky but ideal front rack positioning perfectly set up a dip and drive that earned him a clean and jerk world record that cemented a world record total as well.

Now imagine Vardanyan competing in the super heavyweight weight class where the lightest qualifying lifter could be 27.5kg heavier than the heaviest light heavyweight. Watching Yurik perform his world record snatch and clean and jerk, while still beautiful in their own right, would be like using a golden spoon when wooden fig leaf spoons were available; we know gold is beautiful, but it must be appropriately beautiful to qualify as Plato's Beauty.

Later in those same 1984 Friendship Games, the super heavyweight Alexander Kurlovich's 210kg snatch demonstrated an example of appropriate—yet imperfect—but useful beauty. The snatch is hardly perfect given his left step save. But it would be hard to find a weightlifter, coach, or fan of the sport anywhere who would argue that it was not still a technically beautiful lift. Compare Kurlovich's 210kg snatch with the cleanest, most efficient, and technically flawless snatch we have seen executed in training. Unlike the flawless training snatches we have all seen, Kurlovich might not have performed a snatch that Plato might imagine existing in the realm of the Forms, but his snatch usefully helped Kurlovich earn a silver medal in Varna.

Unfortunately for Kurlovich, Anatoly Pisarenko quickly demonstrated the third type of Beauty that Socrates associates with goodness. Kurlovich's 210kg snatch was 10kg more than Pisarenko's 200kg snatch. Combined with Kurlovich's 252.5kg clean and jerk, his 462.5kg total placed him first in the super heavyweight gold medal slot. In that moment in time and space Pisarenko needed exactly the 265kg clean and jerk he performed to best

Kurlovich with a 465kg total, securing Pisarenko the gold medal.[87] Again, while not technically flawless, Pisarenko's 265kg clean and jerk was exactly what he needed to realize the final goal of every professional weightlifter. Not only was the 265kg the weight Pisarenko needed to win a gold medal, it was the most weight ever cleaned and jerked in competition; a world record that would stand until Leonid Taranenko bested it by 1kg for a 266kg clean and jerk in the Samboy Chips Cup in Australia in 1988. If we agree with Socrates that Beauty must bear some relationship to the good, then we must further agree that a beautiful lift must be one that fulfills the purpose of weightlifting *if* the purpose of weightlifting is to perform a good, white light lift.

This is where Socrates' theory of Beauty diverges from Plato's philosophy of the realm of the Forms. In the realm of the Forms, the most perfect version of anything only exists in the realm of the Forms, not here on Earth where we can see it or touch it.[88] In the case of Beauty, however, Socrates and Hippias seem to agree that some thing's realness allows it to share in the appropriateness, usefulness, and goodness that Socrates says are attributes of beautiful things. Pisarenko's 265kg clean and jerk, then, is a clear example of Beauty in that it may not be the clean and jerk Plato would imagine in the realm of the Forms, but it was appropriate (it was performed at the right time and in the right place) it was useful (it was a weight needed to win the competition) and it was good (it was the heaviest weight ever lifted in a competition).

Thus, we see that one weightlifting competition, the 1984 Friendship Games in Varna, Bulgaria, featured some truly Platonically Beautiful snatches and clean and jerks. The light heavyweight Vardanyan demonstrated that a weight need not be the heaviest ever lifted by any human in any competition to still be technically beautiful and heavy enough to earn him a world record appropriate for his weight class before Alexander Kurlovich took a technically imperfect step in order to save a beautiful snatch, vaulting him into first place in the super heavyweight weight class; a finish that would have held up had Anatoly Pisarenko not executed the greatest lift in history to set his own world records and win gold.

Understanding these various types of Beauty—appropriate, useful, and usefully good—seems almost as Herculean as Pisarenko's 265kg clean and jerk itself. A flawlessly executed world record in one weight class may not seem very impressive when thrown into the mix of the heavier, non-world record setting lifts more easily made in a higher weight class. But a technically inefficient lift might still appear as beautiful as that flawless lower weight if it usefully catapults the heavier lift closer to his ultimate goal of winning a competition. In the end, though, that beautiful lift, too, may be defeated by a movement that encapsulates everything the sport is about: the heaviest weight ever lifted at any time in any competition setting that required it. The *Greater Hippias* dialogue ends, as many of Plato's do, with its participants not completely in agreement or even truly certain of what they agree and disagree on. And our inquiry may end much like the *Greater Hippias* itself, quoting Socrates, saying that he finally understands an old proverb: that beautiful things are difficult.[89]

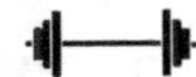

On Dissent: Dismissing the Doubter and Satisfying the Skeptic

Skepticism is fundamentally different from most types of doubt.[90] Doubters may temporarily lack a belief that a proposition is true where Skeptics argue that we cannot know anything for certain. The sophist Gorgias, for example, proposed that nothing exists at all, that even if something did exist, we could not know of its existence, and even if we granted that a single person could know of something's existence, that person could not communicate that knowledge to any other person.[91] Gorgias was a sort of proto-Skeptic who formulated his doubts about knowledge before more organized schools of Skepticism were created.

One such school, Pyrrhonism, was founded by the Greek philosopher, Pyrrho of Elis, in the 4th century BC. Pyrrho's stance on knowledge was softer than Gorgias's; instead of theorizing that nothing exists at all, Pyrrho suggested we simply have no sound reason for preferring one course of action over another. As mentioned in "On Aesthetics: Plato and Pisarenko's Beautiful Lifts," original sources are sometimes hard to find when researching and writing about ancient philosophy. And this is especially true when discussing Pyrrho because, as philosopher and historian of philosophy, Bertrand Russell humorously points out, Pyrrho "very wisely wrote no books."[92] Most of what we know of Pyrrho's philosophy comes from his pupil, Timon of Phlius and one of Pyrrho's detractors, Aristocles of Messene.

In his 1st century history of philosophy, Aristocles paraphrased Timon's summary of Pyrrho, saying that the Skeptic "declared all things to be equally indifferent, indeterminate, and unjudged, and that for that reason neither our senses nor our opinions are reliably true or false. And so we ought not to trust them but should be without opinion, unbiased, and unshaken, saying about each thing that it no more is than is not, or both is and is not, or neither is nor is not."[93] While it is easy to interpret Pyrrho's propositions as claims about what we can or cannot believe, his propositions are also interpretable as propositions about what we should or should not believe.

In his analysis of Aristocles, Timon, and Pyrrho, Professor James Warren carefully details the distinction between Pyrrho as an epistemologist and Pyrrho as a moral philosopher.[94] Warren finds that "there is little reason to think that he...was particularly interested in epistemology at all."[95] Warren instead makes the case for Pyrrho as a moral philosopher concerned with whether things are good or bad and, more specifically, how we can live well. If Pyrrho's teachings are to be understood as an inquiry into living well, his method of instruction still relies heavily on how we might come to know what is good and what is bad.

When searching for means to a happy, well-lived life, Pyrrho argues we must look at three things: how things are, how we should feel about them, and what the result of those two answers will be. Given Pyrrho's theory that all things are equally indifferent and indeterminate, the central philosophy of Pyrrhonian Skepticism, then, is that in order to achieve happiness we must suspend judgment about things we feel we know to be true.[96] It is not so much the case that Pyrrho makes a claim about how the world is or is not so much as he makes a claim that the good is unknowable and, because of that, we should suspend our judgments about the world.

Where most philosophical systems work to acquire new knowledge, the Skeptics organized their philosophy around focusing on whether we can or cannot know anything at all. As Russell frames Pyrrho's skepticism, "there was not much that was new in his doctrine, beyond a certain systematizing and formalizing of older doubts."[97] But this systematic formalizing of older doubts is exactly what distinguishes Skeptics from mere doubters. Where one who holds doubts about a proposition may express reservations, saying *I am not sure*, the Skeptic more adamantly holds *I cannot be sure.*

This position finds a disagreeable partner proposition in the first line of the first book of Aristotle's *Metaphysica*: "All men by nature desire to know."[98] Aristotle's evidence for this claim is "the delight we take in our senses."[99] Epicurus, Aristotle's and Pyrrho's contemporary and fellow Greek, was an empiricist who believed that the only reliable way we can know about the world is what we take in through exactly such senses. Epicurus might respond to the Skeptic's suggestion that because we cannot know whether anything is true, we should suspend judgment about such things, by arguing instead that we can at least know that the information we gather about the world through our senses is true. It is only the judgments about that information that might be true or not.[100] The problem with heavily weighting such evidence is that, if every person takes in the world through his or her senses and uses that sensory input to construct a worldview, if there is even a subtle difference in each perception, all incoming sense perception and—and therefore beliefs about the world—could be both true and false.[101] If a person suffering from color deficiency senses that a shirt is green while a person without a color deficiency senses that the same shirt is red, then we would not be able to truly say either person is right or is wrong. Remember that for these reasons Pyrrho supposedly argued that neither our senses nor our opinions are reliably true or false.[102]

To further build on these theories of knowledge Aristotle, in his *Analytica Posteriora*, contends that "some hold that, owing to the necessity of knowing the primary premises, there is no scientific knowledge."[103] Those holding such a belief, then, may require a demonstration of every proposition in order to get to the bottom of everything. Further, Aristotle reasonably points out, there would be no satisfaction if a proposition is demonstrated to be true, for the Skeptic might then argue that such a demonstration would simply lead to a more fundamental proposition that would necessitate yet another demonstration in order to prove that proposition's truth or falsity.[104] Aristotle finally argues that, even if we were to find some primary proposition at the bottom of all of these satisfactorily demonstrated propositions, the primary proposition might be "unknowable because incapable of demonstration," ultimately leaving the Skeptic still unsatisfied.[105] A second school of Skeptics might concede that truths do exist but that all truths must be demonstrable. Therefore, anything that cannot be demonstrated is not a truth.[106] In either case, there is simply not enough time, nor enough resources, to provide adequate demonstrations for every proposition such that a Skeptic of either school would be able to function in the world if he believed, as Pyrrho suggested, that every proposition is equally true and untrue.

The field of philosophy dealing with gaining knowledge of the world through experience is called empiricism. While empiricism has evolved and fragmented into numerous sub-schools throughout history, empiricists like Epicurus and Aristotle generally hold that if knowledge can be gained at all, it is through our sensory experiences—hearing, seeing, smelling, touching, and tasting—that we are able to construct a fundamental understanding of how the world works. In other words, empiricism does not hold that our senses truthfully provide us with information about the world; only that if we are able to gather truthful information about the world, we can only do it through our senses. Given what we have learned about the logical paradoxes Zeno taught us, Epictetus's instruction on the limits of reason, and Pyrrho's worries about the likelihood of a proposition being true or untrue, empiricism at least offers us a way of learning about the world that makes some intuitive sense.

While empiricism was not a fully formed doctrine of philosophy in Ancient Greece or Rome, many ancient philosophers offered empiricist ideas as we have now come to understand them in light of the school's development in more recent history. Heraclitus, for example, says that "the things that can be seen, heard, and learned are what I prize the most."[107] Aristotle, working to show the importance of understanding primary causes admits that "evidently we have to acquire knowledge of the original causes (for we say we know each thing only when we think we recognize its first cause), and causes are spoken of in four senses."[108] In another of his books he more formally proposes that "(1) no one can learn or understand anything in the absence of sense, and (2) when the mind is actively aware of anything it is necessarily aware of it along with an image."[109] Aristotle appears to agree that, even if what we can know about the world comes from our senses, our senses do not necessarily provide us with a reliable mapping of the world, acknowledging that "Regarding the nature of truth, we must maintain that not everything which appears is true."[110] He carefully distinguishes that "even if sensation—at least of the object peculiar to the sense in question—is not false...appearance is not the same as sensation."[111]

This sort of merger between the sensible and the rational seems at first glance to be somewhat contradictory. Are we to rely on our senses, the appearance of which may deceive us? Or are we to rely on our rationality and logic, the products of which may sometimes be absurd? Here again we find some value in the fundamental proposition of Skepticism: if we cannot reliably know the truth or falsity of a given proposition, we should suspend judgment about that proposition. As Sextus Empiricus puts it, the Skeptics were not trying to obtain knowledge; they were simply trying to find a way to be happy with their opinions and the best they could manage was to not believe anything.[112] On Aristotle's view we find a sort of happy medium; a proposal that we can at least know about the world by what we can gather of it through our senses, but that we must also guard against passive acceptance of what is mere appearance and instead employ a sort of rational and logical screening of what we hear, see, smell, touch, and taste.

For example, there are certainly things upon which all people with the adequate sense perception must agree; for example, whether a 100kg snatch went up or whether it did not. However, there may still be disagreements about whether a left elbow was fully locked out, or whether a clean and jerk was properly held overhead before a down signal was offered, but those differences are measurable in subjective, rather than objective degrees: the truth of the matter exists factually but is interpreted individually. And, to guard against passive acceptance of these subjective differences, most weightlifting competitions feature a three-judge panel along with a five-member jury who may review the judging panel's decision. These layers of review are designed to ensure that some subjective viewpoint does not on its own affect a competition's results.

Whether we are conversing with those who claim that Olympic weightlifting is too dangerous, that a particular coaching method is ineffective, or that championship level feats of physical strength are even possible, what Pyrrho, Timon, Epicurus, Heraclitus, and Aristotle combine to give us is a reasonable way to persuade someone who doubts the validity of some claim we might make. Calhoon and Fry's paper on injury rates and the paper by Junge, et al on sports injuries in the 2008 Olympic games, discussed in detail in "On Embracing Stoicism Through Injury and Triumph" are demonstrative pieces of empirical data that show the relative safety of snatching and clean and jerking. Similarly, the abundance of video footage recorded in training halls and at local, national, and international level competitions provide evidence of otherwise unbelievable displays of human strength achievements. Even with this video evidence, taken together with less convincing but still detailed record keeping and word-of-mouth testimony, Aristotle's distinction between sensation and appearance provides a relevant cautionary tale.

Whether it is simply retail luck or an orchestrated sales tactic we benefit from the fact that most weightlifting plate makers and sellers tend to make similarly weighted bumpers the same colors as other companies make them. Plates measured in kilograms are usually red if they weigh 25kg, blue if 20kg, yellow if 15kg, green if 10kg, white if 5kg. Smaller "change plates" weighing 10% of their larger counterparts are correspondingly colored. A 2.5kg plate is similarly red. A 2kg plate is similarly blue and so on. Plates measured in pounds enjoy the same color scheme for 55, 45, 35, and 25 pounds, respectively.

Therefore, if we see a video of Li Wenwen at the 2019 World Weightlifting Championships in Pattaya, Thailand holding a bar with each side loaded with three full-sized red plates, one small white and one small red plate, a collar, a mini white plate outside the collar, we can be sure that she had just completed a world record 186kg clean and jerk.

Pyrrho is right to be concerned that without any additional information the proposal *Li Wenwen lifted a world record 186kg clean and jerk in Pattaya, Thailand* is just as likely to be false as it is to be true. But we can take a lot of pieces of information into account when determining the validity of the statement. Who told us about the lift? If it was a person we had never met before who had no known history of weightlifting knowledge then we may be neutral about the proposition's validity. If it was said by a known liar seeking to spread chaos among the weightlifting community, then the proposition is more likely to be false. But if we were told about the lift by one of the judges who gave Wenwen a white light in Pattaya, it is much more likely that the statement is true. Furthermore, we can seek out and watch a video recording of the lift, identify the color scheme of the plates, and do the math ourselves to determine how much weight is on the bar. And given the numbers we will see on the screen and the International Weightlifting Federation's certification process undergone by the platemaker, Eleiko, we can unsuspend our judgment and reasonably rely on our senses to believe that Wenwen did, in fact, lift a world record 186kg clean and jerk in Pattaya, Thailand. We used our senses to take in information and used our reasoning to refine that input by determining that we did not see just the *appearance* of a lift: instead, we performed a sort of Aristotelian empirical verification to satisfy the skeptic in us.

A more challenging skeptic to satisfy is one who does not believe that some prospective coach will be able to provide meaningful instruction to a prospective athlete or client. In the case of Wenwen's world record we have a past event that, having occurred, can be replayed in order to persuade a skeptic of its occurrence. In this case, however, we have to find a way to persuade the skeptic that a future event will occur; that the coach will offer a client instruction that will improve, in some meaningful manner, that client's ability to snatch or clean and jerk. Again, we can turn to Aristotle for help.

In yet another of his books, *Analytica Priora*, Aristotle establishes the first full treatment of a system of logic. He specifically develops a system of analysis called deductive reasoning known as syllogism. Aristotle defines a syllogism as "discourse in which, certain things being stated, something other than what is stated follows of necessity from their being so."[113] These syllogisms start with a major premise and a minor premise and end with a conclusion with nothing more than a logical assumption in between. For Aristotle, a syllogism goes like this: Socrates is a man, man is mortal, therefore Socrates is mortal. Aristotle was the first to provide a formula for reasoning through making hypotheses based on their likenesses to similar things.[114] When working to persuade a skeptic that a coach is well-suited for a client's needs, syllogisms serve as a tool useful for helping us overcome a skeptic's suspended judgments about whether that coach is, in fact, well-suited for the task: Coach A provided instruction for Weightlifter B and Weightlifter B is a successful weightlifter. Therefore, Coach A provided Weightlifter B with instruction that made Weightlifter B a successful weightlifter. This loosely formulated piece of logic can be supported even further by demonstrating the probability that each premise and the conclusion is true.[115] Here, we turn to a fifth of Aristotle's books to strengthen our persuasive toolkit.

In *Rhetorica*, Aristotle says that *enthymemes* "are the substance of rhetorical persuasion."[116] He defines an *enthymeme* as "a syllogism starting from probabilities or signs."[117] He differentiates between probabilities and signs, teaching that "a probability is a generally approved proposition: what men know to happen or not to happen, to be or not to be, for the most part thus and thus" while a sign "means a demonstrative proposition necessary or generally approved."[118] While Aristotle did not coin the term, he more or less reframed our understanding of an *enthymeme* to be a method of persuasion that assumes certain premises based on probabilities or signs. Rather than offer a full syllogism: Socrates is a man, man is mortal, therefore Socrates is mortal, the *enthymeme* might go: Socrates is mortal because he is a man.

Given all that we know about Skeptics—that they do not believe any proposition is more or less likely to be true or untrue, and given what we know about the time-consuming nature of demonstrating all propositions to all Skeptics, we can usefully employ Aristotle's *enthymeme* when persuading a skeptic that a coach's instruction is a valuable method of obtaining useful knowledge that can be utilized to make a prospective client a better weightlifter. None of this is to say that a coach's ability to effectively pass on information or instruction should be simply assumed by any prospective client. But we should feel comfortable suggesting that, rather than needing to demonstrate every proposition a coach might make to a prospective client— e.g., here is how I can make you stronger, here is how I can make you faster, here is how I can make you more technically proficient, specifically how I can improve your third pull under the bar—if a coach has enough experience under her belt and has enough of a body of work to rely on, then it is likely that coach enjoys the sort of skill set that will also help her help the next weightlifter.

Even a Skeptic should be able to withdraw his suspension of judgment when the probability that weightlifting is a sport that can be safely participated in, that a specific weight was lifted by some specific athlete—in spite of the intuitive unlikelihood of such a marvelous feat—and that there is a coach out there that can improve the power, speed, and quality of movement of athletes of all experience levels, when faced with the chain of demonstration outlined above. That skeptic just needs to encounter the proper method of persuasion. Even Aristotle might be able to convince Pyrrho of all such propositions.

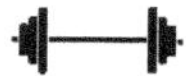

On Refuting the Sophist: Aristotelian Avoidance of the Accidental

In "On Dealing with Dissent: Dismissing the Doubter and Satisfying the Skeptic" we explored Aristotle's syllogisms, philosophy's introduction to a system of formal logic. To refresh, Aristotle defines a syllogism as "discourse in which, certain things being stated, something other than what is stated follows of necessity from their being so."[119] A syllogism contains three parts: two premises and a conclusion. The premises can be thought of propositions, or evidence. And the conclusion is what the propositions, or evidence, show as true based on nothing more than what the propositions, or evidence, purport to be true.

Aristotle immediately distinguishes between a perfect syllogism—one "which needs nothing other than what has been stated to make plain what necessarily follows"—and an imperfect syllogism—one that "needs either one or more propositions, which are indeed the necessary consequences of the terms set down, but have not been expressly stated as premises."[120] More plainly stated, Aristotle's perfect syllogisms do not need to be proved; their terms speak for themselves, while his imperfect syllogisms need some additional explaining.

Although Aristotle himself did not offer this specific example of a syllogism, these two premises (*P1* and *P2*) and a conclusion (C) are the premiere example known by most philosophy students today:

P1: All men are mortal.
P2: Socrates is a man.
C: Socrates is mortal.

Such a syllogism is categorized as perfect because it explains itself. We do not need to dig any deeper than the information that has been provided in order to understand that if *P1* is true and *P2* is true, then *C* must be true. The completeness of this information is what distinguishes Aristotle's perfect syllogisms from his imperfect syllogisms.

In *Analytica Priora* Aristotle offers the following notation as an example of an imperfect syllogism:

> "Let *M* be predicated of no *N*, but all of *O*.
> Since, then, the negative relation is convertible,
> *N* will belong to no *M*: but *M* was assumed to
> belong to all *O*: consequently *N* will belong to
> no *O*."[121]

In plain speak:

P1: No competition snatches are judged during powerlifting competitions.

P2: All competition clean and jerks are performed after competition snatches.

C: Therefore, competition clean and jerks are not performed at powerlifting competitions.

Unlike the perfect syllogism proving Socrates' mortality, this imperfect syllogism requires us to look beyond the explicitly presented information and deduce from *P*1 and *P*2 some impossibility: that if clean and jerks are performed after snatches and there are no snatches performed in powerlifting competitions, then clean and jerks must logically not be performed at powerlifting competitions.

A further note must be considered before we evaluate what we can learn about weightlifting from this piece of ancient philosophy: that of the philosophical distinction between logical *validity* and logical *soundness*. The logical form *P*1 + *P*2 = *C* is a valid logical equation if *P*1, *P*2, and *C* share some common proposition distributed across all three parts. In the above Socrates example *P*1, *P*2, and *C* all share in some common proposition regarding either Socrates, mortality, or both. Crucially, *P*1, *P*2, and *C* do not need to be empirically true in order for the logical equation to be valid. Consider the following example:

> *P*1: Socrates is a duck.
> *P*2: All ducks are immortal.
> *C*: Socrates is immortal.

Socrates was not, empirically speaking, a duck. Nor are all ducks immortal. However, according to Aristotle, the equation is still logical because given the distributed propositions *P*1 + *P*2 does, logically equate to *C*. Never mind Socrates not being a duck and ducks not being immortal. Aristotle deals with numerous methods of identifying and dismantling unsound, but logical, propositions in his work *De Sophisticis Elenchis*, another of his books in the *Organon*.

In addition to his linguistic refutations, all of which deal with language tricks, Aristotle identifies as one of seven non-linguistic refutations *accidental* fallacies.[122] Aristotle proposes that an accidental fallacy occurs when "it is claimed that some attribute belongs to the thing and to its accident."[123] We identify some object or being as being comprised of some series of properties, some of those properties are unique to that object or being, and some are properties shared with other objects or beings. Some unique property of an object may be its serial number; some unique property of a being is its genome sequence. Other properties that may comprise an object or being but are accidental and shared by other objects or beings may be size, age, or educational background. Aristotle had his unique genome sequence and he also studied under Plato. No one in history shared Aristotle's genome sequence but many other philosophers, including Aristonymus and Heraclides of Aenus, also studied under Plato.[124] So while it is logical to say:

> *P*1: Aristotle studied philosophy under Plato.
> *P*2: Plato's philosophy student assassinated Cotys I, ruler of Thrace.
> *C*: Aristotle assassinated Cotys I, ruler of Thrace.

Again, while logically valid, this sequence is an example of Aristotle's fallacy of accident. Aristotle did, in fact, study philosophy under Plato, but so did Heraclides of Aenus, Cotys I's actual assassin.[125]

It is this common, accidental attribute that Aristotle and Heraclides of Aenus share that adds enough ambiguity to *P*1 and *P*2 to make *C* valid within the context of the logical propositions but unsound when evaluated against what actually happened in the world. And where the world is concerned these ambiguities are too frequently exploited and leveraged in order to take advantage of those who may not understand that just because $A = B$, B does not necessarily $= A$.

If we substitute Aristotle with any given weightlifting coach or athlete in the world and Plato's academy with some educational provenance or accomplishment, then Aristotle's *De Sophisticis Elenchis* becomes a sort of handbook for determining who is and who is not worth devoting energy to when trying to improve one's skills and abilities in the barbell sports world. Consider the following:

> *P*1: Coach A won an Olympic weightlifting gold medal.

P2: An Olympic weightlifting gold medal winning coach is the best coach to learn from.

C: Coach A is the best coach to learn from.

Given what we learned from Aristotle's instruction on syllogisms, these two premises lead to a logically valid conclusion. And when some unsuspecting laylifter decides to hire a coach or join a gym, *an Olympic weightlifting gold medalist coaches here!* is an understandably attractive marketing campaign. However, understanding Aristotle's *De Sophisticis Elenchis*, specifically the fallacy of accident, shows that success as a lifter does not necessarily translate to effectiveness as a coach. In the above case *P1* + *P2* may validly equate to *C*, and it may even soundly equate to *C*. However, if it is both a valid and sound logical equation, it is only so accidentally. There is quite likely an overwhelmingly larger number of Olympic gold medalists who would be suboptimal coaches if they chose to transfer from the competitive to the coaching arena. In Aristotelian terms, if Coach A did win an Olympic weightlifting gold medal and Coach A is additionally the best coach to learn from, Coach A is not the best coach to learn from *because of the gold medal win*.

While it can be true—and in many cases is true—that Olympic weightlifting legends like Hossein Rezazadeh and Pyrros Dimas followed up their spectacular competitive careers with impressive coaching tenures, they are not exceptions to Aristotle's rules. Another legend of the sport, Leonid Zhabotynsky, despite dedicating his post-competition career to coaching his nation's military rather than focusing his knowledge and efforts on competitive lifters, underwrote his professional experience and talent with a PhD in pedagogy from the Kharkiv Pedagogical Institute.[126] Waldemar Baszanowski, the five-time World Championship and two-time Olympic gold medalist also bolstered his historical lifting resume by becoming a lecturer at the Polish Academy of Physical Education in addition to coaching the Indonesian national weightlifting team.[127]

If we recall the earlier chapter "On Selecting a Coach: The Systemic Art of Identifying the Sophist" Plato provides, across multiple books, a thorough inquiry into what a sophist is and helped us understand that a virtuous teacher is the one who works to help a student get closer to the truth while a sophist corrupts that same educational journey by interweaving the truth with falsity. It is Aristotle's *De Sophisticis Elenchis* that delineates into a formal logic a useful series of ways to dismantle the sophist's convolution of that which we should want to know for our sake and that which the sophist wants us to know for the sophist's sake. Taking this into account we can view the above equation in this way:

*P*1: Coach A won an Olympic weightlifting gold medal. And she did so due to her dedication to her craft, her relentless pursuit of excellence, and prodigious combination of talent and disciplined hard work.

*P*2: An Olympic weightlifting gold medal winning coach is the best coach to learn from. But Coach A's aptitude for coaching is merely accidental to her gold medal win. In addition to—but not because of—her platform victory, she is also a master communicator with a world-class breadth and depth of knowledge of the intricacies of the sport, its programming, attempt weight openings and increases, and has an ability to understand the needs of her client athletes.

C: Coach A is the best coach to learn from.

On Coaching as a Performance: Aristotelian Categoriae

To the uneducated hearer *I am a powerlifter*, *I am a weightlifter*, and *I lift weights* all seem to tell the same story. To anyone with any tenure in the sport of powerlifting or the sport of weightlifting, each of these three statements outlines varying levels of participation in entirely distinct activities. Similarly, the declarations *I am a weightlifter* and *I am a weightlifting coach* describe two different roles that play a part in the same sport. Fundamentally *powerlifter*, *weightlifter*, *lifter of weights*, and *coach* are discrete terms each referring to a particular definition or description. Each of these terms fits, however neatly or sloppily, into what Aristotle called, simply, *categories*.

In *Categoriae*, another of his six works on logic and dialectic that constitute Aristotle's *Organon*, the philosopher enumerates ten categories into which all fathomable concepts fit. Translation variations notwithstanding, Aristotle's ten categories are as follows:

1. Substance
2. Quantity
3. Quality
4. Relative To
5. Where
6. When
7. Relative Position

8. Having
9. Doing
10. Being Affected

Our primary concern and the focus of our conversation will be with the first four categories: *substance, quantity, relative to,* and *quality.*

Insofar as *substance* goes, Aristotle further divides the category into primary and secondary substances. A primary substance is a particular substance where a secondary substance is more universal. For instance, Aristotle is a particular human who was born in 384 BC in a northeastern Grecian city called Stagira. Aristotle is also a man. Aristotle, *the* 4th century Stagirite may be categorized as a *primary substance* whereas the man*ness* of Aristotle the man, is Aristotle as a *secondary substance.* That which describes Aristotle as a primary substance belongs to Aristotle and Aristotle alone but that which describes Aristotle as a secondary substance is also that which describes all others that can be categorized as that same secondary substance. Aristotle and Lasha Talakhadze, whose existences are separated by roughly two-and-a-half millennia, each fit into the *substance* category—in this case the *secondary substance*—in that they are both some version of *man.* Still, each of them also fits into Aristotle's *primary substance* individually; Aristotle with his Aristotle*ness* and Lasha with his Lasha*ness.*

While Aristotle's treatment of his second category, *quantity,* is a bit involved, the overall concept is really rather simple compared to the rest of the list. Because the idea of some amount of a thing is separate from the thing itself, *quantity*—despite Aristotle's best efforts to the contrary—cannot be intermixed with any other category.[128] Like *substance, quantity* is broken down into a few subcategories: *continuous quantities* like *line, surface, body, time,* and *space* and *discrete quantities* like *number* and *speech.* According to Aristotle everything that fits into every other category fits also into *quantity* given its relation to each subcategory. Where *number* does not describe Aristotle, the *substance* called *man* does. But there being only Aristotle, that *quantity* describes how many Aristotles there are: one.[129]

Aristotle says next that "those things are called relative, which being either said to be *of* something else or *related to* something else, are explained by reference to that other thing."[130] Unlike *substance* and *quantity* this third category *relative* requires two of some instances of another category. Aristotle's example, *superior*, can only be categorized as some thing being *superior* to some other thing. The same is true of *perception* and *knowledge*. Neither concept can stand alone; they can only be conceived of in relation to some other thing: *perception* of some movement and *knowledge* of some fact, for example. Some, though not all *relatives* also have contraries. The contrary of *knowledge* is *ignorance* and the contrary of *superior* is *inferior*. Other relatives like *double* or *triple* do not have any contraries. Additionally, Aristotle points out "that *relatives* can admit of variation of degree." Some thing can be more or less *like* or *unlike* another thing or more or less *equal* or *unequal* to something else.[131]

Finally, for the sake of our discussion, Aristotle says of *quality*—quite vaguely and a bit unhelpfully—that he means "that in virtue of which people are said to be such and such."[132] To clarify the *such and such* Aristotle divides *quality* into a few subcategories: *habits* like "various kinds of knowledge and of virtue," and *dispositions* by which he means "a condition that is easily changed and quickly gives place to its opposite" like hotness and coldness or wellness and illness.[133] Additionally Aristotle suggests that another *quality* is that that makes "men good boxers or runners or healthy or sickly," qualities he claims are inborn capacities.[134] Hardness and softness also fall into this subcategory in virtue of an object's capacity to resist or withstand disintegration. His third class in the *quality* subcategory is "that of affective qualities and affections" such as "sweetness, bitterness, sourness, whiteness, and blackness."[135] And Aristotle's fourth, and final enumerated *quality* subcategory is a thing's figure and shape; "straightness and curvedness" for example.[136]

In classical Aristotelian semi-finality, he admits that "there may be other sorts of quality, but those that are most properly so called have, we may safely say, been enumerated."[137] Crucially, though, Aristotle does further instruct that "qualities admit of variation of degree."[138] A white thing can be more or less white than another thing and a sour thing can be more or less sour than another thing. Also, one white thing can become more or less white by varying degrees across time and space. So, too, can a sour thing become more or less sour than itself at some point in time. So, while Aristotle's categories are presumably exhausted, some categories feature subcategories and degrees of variation within those.

If all of what we know about the universe can fit into some of these categories, then understanding the categories teaches us a great deal about each's contents. In the first sentence of *Categoriae* Aristotle suggests that "things are said to be named *equivocally* when, though they have a common name, the definition corresponding with the same differs for each."[139] Equivocally speaking, if we travel to a Georgian weightlifting facility and point at the world record holding superheavyweight we can say "Lasha Talakhadze" and be just as intelligibly understood as if, while watching a video of that same man's 492kg total performance at the 2021 World Weightlifting Championship in Tashkent, we point at that figure on the screen and say "Lasha Talakhadze." *Lasha Talakhadze* refers to both the human in front of us in Georgia and to the man on the screen snatching 225kg and clean and jerking 267kg.

"On the other hand," Aristotle argues, "things are said to be named *univocally* which have both the name and the definition answer to the name in common."[140] We might then univocally refer to Lasha and fellow Olympian Sarah Robles and say "weightlifter" as both distinct individuals are correctly categorized as participants in the same sport.

Two curious cases emerge, however when we consider the equivocal and univocal references to individuals like Sarah Robles, multi-time Olympic medalist and world champion weightlifter and USA Weightlifting Technical Director and coach, Pyrros Dimas.[141,142] Hardly any fan of the sport would think to correct us if we were to point to both Robles and Dimas and say "weightlifter." Both Robles and Dimas have Olympic Games experience with the former competing in Rio De Janeiro in 2016 and Tokyo in 2020 and the latter in Barcelona, Atlanta, Sydney, and Athens in 1992, 1996, 2000, and 2004 respectively. Both individuals can boast Olympic medals in their trophy cases with Robles earning bronze in both 2016 and 2020 and Dimas golds in 1992, 1996, and 2000 and a bronze in 2004. Robles and Dimas also each have at least one first-place podium appearance at a World Weightlifting Championship with the American born earning her gold in Anaheim in 2017 and the Albanian capturing three in Melbourne, Guangzhou, and Lathi in 1993, 1995, and 1998. As of this writing, however, only one of the two, Sarah Robles, is an active participant in the sport called Olympic Weightlifting. Pyrros Dimas, a fixture of the sport for four decades, is no longer competitive. At least not on a platform.

Are we making an Aristotelian miscategorization, then, if we refer to both Robles and Dimas as *weightlifter* if only one of the individuals is a currently competitive member of the sport? Recalling Aristotle's *substance*—specifically his *secondary substance*—because that which describes all of those who fit into the category *weightlifter* might apply to more than one individual means more than one individual can be accurately called a weightlifter. We need not worry that only one being can be categorized as a weightlifter because Aristotle instructs that both Robles and Dimas can be categorized as weightlifters when discussing the category *quantity*; specifically, the subcategory *number*—i.e. the *quantity* of intelligibles that share in the quality of *weightlifter* is more than one because both Sarah Robles the woman and Pyrros Dimas the man share in what refers to *weightlifter*.

Furthermore, while we discussed Plato's Theory of Forms and the aesthetic beauty that might organize what it is to be the theoretically ideal weightlifter, Aristotle's *relative to* category opens the admission gates to a variety of *weightlifter* referents. Picture and video evidence documentation provide proof that both Robles and Dimas have lifted barbells off the ground and placed them overhead in either one smooth motion or in two separate and distinct movements that comprise the snatch and the clean and jerk.

Irrespective of the kilogram weight of the barbells and bumper plates both individuals may thereby be categorized as weightlifters. Is this alone enough for each to qualify as a weightlifter or does the amount of weight lifted or time period over which each's tenure endured qualify or disqualify either or both of them as a weightlifter or non-weightlifter?

To satisfy this line of inquiry we can rely on the *relative to* category as a hybrid reference to Aristotle's variations of degrees.[143] Just as a barbell's knurling may be less *shiny* after it's ten thousandth pull off the platform, Dimas may be less *weightlifter* now—per kilo lifted over some period of time— than he was when he snatched 180kg and clean and jerked 213kg in Atlanta in 1996, setting two world records in the process.[144] Likewise, when Robles snatched 128kg and clean and jerked 154kg for a 282kg total in the Tokyo Olympics in 2021 we cannot say she was a lesser lifter than she was when she snatched 126kg and clean and jerked 160kg for a 286kg total in the 2016 Olympics in Rio de Janeiro. In both performances, Robles earned a bronze medal.

From all of this we can take away a few crucial lessons. First, the category *weightlifter* is quite an umbrella. What the actual definition is—one who has performed a single lifetime rep of one or both of the sport's required movements or one who snatches and clean and jerks competitively, or some other agreed upon set of conditions—is important but it is more important to understand that *weightlifter*, as a category, can mean a lot of things and many, many individuals can fit into that mold. A septuagenarian grandmother and a world record holder, so long as both individuals satisfy that set of conditions, are both weightlifters. The strongest woman in the world and the history's winningest Olympian do not, if they do not satisfy the same set of conditions. Second, an individual can be categorized in many different ways. Sarah Robles is an American, and she is a weightlifter, and she is an Olympic medalist. Pyrros Dimas is an Albanian-born Greek, and he is a weightlifter, and he is an Olympic medalist. Third, within each category the categorized can vary by degree and in relation to another. If weightlifter A snatches 200kg and weightlifter B snatches

5kg, the strength difference between the two lifters does not qualify or disqualify one or the other as a weightlifter, only their satisfaction of the set of conditions that defines *weightlifter*.

Now that we understand the descriptive—how the language is used—we can work out the prescriptive—how we should use it.

In spite of Aristotle's instruction, it is sometimes difficult to view the similarities between two things that effectively function as the flipsides of a single coin. In weightlifting we often talk about things in terms of their differences or what makes them distinct. This lift, that lift, this rep of that set, or the athlete's role versus the coach's role. While recognizing the unique aspects of lifts, programs, and individuals permits us to analyze various attributes of each, in turn helping us improve upon those attributes, sometimes seeking out what makes one like the other more efficiently guides our perfection-seeking athletic analysis.

As discussed in *Categoriae* one way to describe something is to say that it is more or less like some other thing in the same category. A snatch is like a clean and jerk in that each of them is an Olympic weightlifting movement, but the movements are not alike in that a snatch is a single fluid movement of the barbell from the floor to the overhead position while a clean and jerk features separate movements from the floor to the shoulders and then the shoulders to the overhead position. A single repetition is like a single set in that both are elements of a larger compilation of movements. But a single repetition must be schemed for a percentage of how many reps will be performed in a set where a set must be weighed against the total number of sets in a workout in the instant movement as well as sets of other movements. And a coach and an athlete are similar in that they are the two central figures in the sport of weightlifting but strikingly dissimilar in that the athlete moves the bar while the coach moves the athlete. None of these observations is meant to be taken in any way as a valuation. A snatch is not worth more than a clean and jerk and neither the single repetition nor whole set is more important than the other. For our purposes we will focus on what is the most valuable of all of these relationships:

that of the coach and the athlete. Not only is neither more important than the other—outside of some unheard of hyperathlete who may someday win Olympic gold without the benefit of a coach's guidance—it is probably the relationship best improved upon by focusing on the common attributes each individual shares, rather than focusing specifically on what makes each role unique.

It is not unreasonable to say that there is probably no clearer relationship distinction in athletics than that between an athlete and a coach. A lift is a lift and a movement is a movement but only one individual has her hands on the bar while the other is offering instruction, encouragement, or admonishment from the sideline. This is not to say that only the athlete participates in the glory of victory or the gloom of failure. Only the weightlifter will know how the bar feels overhead when the cameras are flashing and the crowd is cheering. But in that moment the coach's smile may be bigger than the lifter's. Conversely, everyone who has ever even so much as helped a fellow athlete navigate the treacheries of the obstacle course that is determining opening lift numbers and weight jumps throughout a session knows well the shared feeling of disappointment when the one who pulls the bar fails to achieve at least two white lights. The coach knows just as well the despair that accompanies the missed footwork that leads to the pressed out jerk when the athlete fails to post a total. Because while the athlete may rest after the meet knowing she did all she could and that she just did not have what it took to be successful that day, the coach will turn over in his head the disturbing thought that maybe he simply failed to better instruct the athlete that the back foot must turn inward in order to accommodate the overhead load.

Each of these roles, however, share multiple conditions of one very specific Aristotelian category: *performer*. Both coach and athlete have a task they must perform in order to be called either coach or athlete. The coach must offer instruction to the athlete and the athlete must lift the bar in a prescribed manner. Thus, the actual distinction lies not in which of the pair does the performing, but in the role each performer is to play. One of the individuals performs on a platform, a court, or a field. The other individual performs on the sideline and in the trenches of academia. Despite the difference in arena, both coach and athlete share enough common traits that their coordination in the *performer* category requires further consideration.

In the first place we can say that the same philosophical mechanisms that allow us to describe something in terms of its similarity to something else, in order to make a value statement, also allow us to prescribe ways to improve the way a coach approaches his task by describing coaching *as a performance*.

Take a moment to consider a set of conditions that must be met in order for one to be filed away in the category *performer*: *one who performs* to be sure, and now what conditions must be met to satisfy *performance*?

- the carrying out of an action
- the delivery of a service
- the implementation of a plan
- the discharge of a duty

Simply stated a *performance*, as a verb, is some action done in furtherance of some goal. A *performer*, then, is the individual undertaking that action. In such a category the action or goal is not itself relevant. In the instant inquiry the lifter must lift, and the coach must coach. And, if our discussion of Plato's Theory of Forms teaches us anything, it is that we can conceive of an ideal lifter and an ideal coach. Where we analyzed what the ideal lifter may be in "On Aesthetics: Plato and Pisarenko's Beautiful Lifts" and "On Perfection: Platonism and Competition" there is some work to be done to ascertain the conditions that categorize the ideal coach.

When a coach is performing, he is playing a role: supporter, teacher, theoretician. When an athlete is performing, she is playing a role: weightlifter, competitor, entertainer. And if the ultimate function of a performer is to best some other performer in competition, then both coach and athlete must fulfill their intended function as close to optimally as possible.[145] In every competition, physical or otherwise, there is one element of performance that must always be maximized: efficiency.

For an athlete, maximizing efficiency tends to be a relatively straightforward process. For a weightlifter, keeping the barbell close to the body will maximize mechanical advantage and will allow a larger weight to be moved with minimal force. Maximizing this efficiency will allow an overall weaker athlete to lift bigger weights than a stronger athlete, provided the stronger athlete does not maximize her own mechanical advantage.

For a coach, maximizing efficiency can be more complicated. For an athlete to perform efficiently, she must master complex biomechanical relationships both within herself and without. For a coach to perform efficiently, he must understand and master complex biomechanical *and* psychological relationships. And, like most relationships, mastery begins within oneself.

Familiar is the scene: the reddened face and bulbous veins, the heightened vocal volume and vocabulary limited to a few four-letter words. The athlete's head down while her hands are on her hips, the coach screaming some usually obvious suggestion for how the athlete can get it right the next time. Sometimes the athlete just needs a little reminder of the seriousness of some aspect of the movement, and, in such cases, a little vocal motivation is due and proper. But to truly maximize a coach's effectiveness in conveying that motivation, he must master his own efficiency *as a performer.*

Of all of the moving parts in a coach/athlete relationship, understanding what motivates an athlete is key to unlocking all the others. That scene described is only all-too familiar because it is rarely the most effective method of communication. Unfortunately, many coaches fail to recognize that the highway is not the only alternative to their way. When was the precedent set that an athlete must conform to a coach's teaching style, but a coach owes no duty to the athlete to tailor his method to the individual seeking guidance?

It makes sense that an athlete seeking a coach exercises some amount of discretion; there are certainly more or less knowledgeable coaches and the coach who understands his respective field is more valuable than the coach who has barely scratched the surface of the endeavor. But that does not seem to be a reason that the coach must not further his performance ability by maximizing his understanding of how to most effectively impart that knowledge. All the information in the world is worthless if a coach is unable to maximize his teaching advantage in order to most efficiently convey knowledge to his athlete.[146] If it is a suboptimal mechanical advantage that lessens an athlete's ability to overcome an otherwise superior athletic competitor, then a coach's suboptimal teaching advantage likewise lessens his ability to overcome an otherwise superior coaching competitor.

It is not enough for a coach to think like a coach. For a coach to truly maximize his teaching advantage, he must think like an athlete. A coach's need to overcome inefficiencies tends not to manifest itself in a failure to comprehend the biomechanical or strategic advantages of a given athletic or mental competition. More likely it is an inability to find effective means of communication that hampers a coach's teaching advantage. An athlete's mechanical advantage lies in biomechanics; a coach's teaching advantage lies in his philosophy.

It is not enough for a coach to know the way to describe an advantageous approach to competition. He must be like the athlete in adapting to strategies that help him overcome obstacles to efficiency. He must approach coaching as a technique that needs constant refinement and philosophical mastery; not only as a well of knowledge that is to be filled to the brim and left for the athlete to draw from. Performers understand that there is no completion. Medals and trophies are a way to keep score and the athlete who performs well enough to earn the highest score is the best. But performers understand that there is no such thing as perfection. There is only better or worse; and constant betterment is the only path to victory. In the same way, a coach must understand that there is no such thing as perfection. There is only better or worse and an inability to recognize deficiencies is a sure way to guarantee failure.

Due to the complex relationships between coach and athlete, athlete and biomechanical mastery, biomechanical mastery and understanding, and understanding imparting of knowledge, the concept of coaching as a performance presents itself as a seemingly infinite series of moving parts. This is not to say that coaching is harder than competing; only that coaching is not so simple a task as learning about a topic and passing on that knowledge to an athlete in whatever manner the instructor sees fit.

To be truly effective, a coach must approach his task with the same focus on efficiency as an athlete. A coach cannot attempt to instruct his athletes with a narrow-minded approach; not because his approach may be wrong, but because it may not be as right as it could be. And it is a coach's focus on maximizing his teaching advantage that allows him to perform with maximal efficiency in the same way a weightlifter approaches a heavily loaded barbell. Physics plays a pivotal role in weightlifting, but it is not the only role. Psychological mastery also plays a role. While all of the psychological mastery in the world will not allow humans to raise thousands of pounds over their heads without the aid of machinery or run a sub-two-minute mile, it is the mental approach to a task that provides an athlete a competitive advantage over a less mentally sound adversary, all biomechanical factors being equal. It is similarly true that the more informed coach is going to have an advantage over a lesser informed coach, but it is the coach who is able to impart a greater amount of knowledge to his athlete who is going to be more successful. And for a coach to truly perform at the highest level—his ability to approach his goal of imparting the greatest amount of knowledge in the most efficient manner—he must approach his task not only as a coach, but as a performer.

Epilogue: On Socratic Savage Strength

*"He no longer makes any use of persuasion but
bulls his way through every situation by force and
savagery like a wild animal, living in ignorance
and stupidity without either rhythm or grace."*[147]

In what may appear to be a bit of a departure from the central theme of a project called *Plato's Barbell*, Plato himself—through his trusted mouthpiece, Socrates—unintentionally offers us an approach to the sport that most of this book seems to argue against: that the surest path to weightlifting success is a complete disregard for any academic undertaking not related to the sport itself.

Where cautious and conservative or holistic and well-rounded are fine approaches to many an endeavor, the acquisition of the savage strength required to win gold is not such an endeavor. This idea is not so much a hard and fast rule as much as it is an ongoing observation. When observing the strongest men and women in the world actual training philosophies and programming theories may vary. One constant, however, is invariably present in each and every athlete: a noticeable focusing on nothing other than the task at hand.

In Book III of Plato's *Republic* Socrates discusses with Glaucon the values and drawbacks of various approaches to education. Socrates and

Glaucon agree that those who are naturally well endowed in body and soul are better off than those whose bodies are naturally unhealthy or incurably evil. They further agree that a person who pursues an education in music and poetry in moderation will pursue physical training in moderation as well. Such individuals will work at physical exercise to arouse their spirited nature rather than to acquire the sort of physical strength for which athletes diet and labor.

To prove his point Socrates asks Glaucon if Glaucon has noticed the effect that a lifetime of physical training has on a person when not rounded out by music or poetry and, conversely, a lifetime of music and poetry when not balanced with physical training. When Glaucon asks Socrates to explain, Socrates argues that a dedication to physical training, without being moderated by the arts, leads to "savagery and toughness" while the opposite life leads to "softness and overcultivation."[148]

I learned about the art of weightlifting in the back of a dusty granite shop in an industrial strip mall in Southern Nevada. I was never in the gym to become a world champion or an Olympian but, to a man, everyone else there was. I was surrounded by some of the best lifters and smartest minds in the sport and I soaked up every piece of data that flew my way. There was no music. There was frequently very little conversation. There were only Ironmind VHS tapes and training hall videos played on repeat.

After a few years immersing myself in the world of barbell sports in various gyms, competitions, and seminars I realized that among the many differences between the sort of top-tier athletes from that dusty old off-the-beaten-path gym and the average barbell lifter, one crucial difference mattered more than any other: not only did the top athletes *want* championship level strength more, they had no reservations about *getting it*. This is not to say that every rep and every set the top-level athletes performed was designed to go

A Note on the Sources

A link to purchase all of these sources is available at platosbarbell.com:

All references to Epictetus are taken from *The Stoic and Epicurean Philosophers* edited by W.J. Oates, published by the *Modern Library*.

All references to Epicurus are taken from *The Stoic and Epicurean Philosophers* edited by W.J. Oates, published by the *Modern Library*.

All references to Heraclitus's fragments can be found at http://www.heraclitusfragments.com, indexed by the corresponding Diels-Kranz numbers (last referenced 10/17/2023).

All references to Daedelus and Icarus are taken from Ovid's *Metamorphosis*, Book VIII translated by Frank Justus Miller, published by Harvard University Press for the Loeb Classical Library.

All references to Parmenides' fragments can be found at https://plato.stanford.edu/entries/parmenides/ with direct links to the corresponding Diels-Kranz numbers (last referenced 10/17/2023).

All references to Plato's writings are taken from *Plato: Complete Works* edited by John M. Cooper, published by Hackett Publishing Company.

All references to biographies found in Plutarch's Lives are taken from *Plutarch's Lives Volume I* translated by John Dryden and revised by A.H. Clough, published by the *Modern Library*.

Other Books

History of Western Philosophy by Bertrand Russell

How Architecture Works: A Humanist's Toolkit by Witold Rybczynski, published by Farrar, Straus, and Giroux (2014)

The Story of Philosophy by Will Durant, published by Simon & Schuster (1967)

The Story of Athens: The Fragments of the Local Chronicles of Attika by Philip Harding

De Corpore by Thomas Hobbes

Lives of the Eminent Philosophers by Diogenes Laertius, translated by Pamela Mensch

Outlines of Pyrrhonism by Sexuts Empiricus, translated by R.G. Bury

---

[1] Epictetus, *Discourses*, Book II, Chapter XI

[2] Ibid.

[3] Ibid.

[4] When discussing Plato, it is useful to use upper case letters when mentioning the Platonic description of something's form, e.g., the upper-case *F* Form is man, while the lower-case *f* form is a man.

[5] Dr. Alexander Nehamas offers a different perspective on whether Plato values a thing's Form as more perfect than its sensible particular, arguing that—at least in some cases—a particular suffers not from *imperfection* so much as *incapacity*. See Nehamas, A. (1975). Plato on the Imperfection of the Sensible World. *American Philosophical Quarterly*, *12*(2), 105–117. http://www.jstor.org/stable/20009565

[6] Most of what these ideas are concerned with are physical instantiations of a Form or Idea, but Plato also discusses the Ideal versions of nonphysical Forms like Beauty (*Symposium* 211) and Justice (*Phaedo* 65d). We use *sensible* to refer to that which can be reached by our senses and is not only theoretical like that which is in the realm of the Forms.

[7] *Cratylus* 389c

[8] Ibid.

[9] The physicalized version of its more perfect form can be called—rather counterintuitively—its idea, from the Greek εἶδος, used to describe something's viewable outward appearance.

[10] *Theaetetus* 185c

[11] *Republic VII* 514

[12] *Republic VII* 518c

[13] *Republic VII* 518e

[14] *Republic VII* 517c

[15] This may not be true of the coach is seeking something other than to impart true knowledge of the sport. Coaches motivated by financial benefit or some other material gain are more likely to attempt to appease their athletes than coaches who truly wish to see their athletes succeed in the sport. See the chapter "On Selecting a Coach: The Systemic Art of Identifying the Sophist" for more.

[16] In the 21st century alone, the 2020 Olympic Games saw Rahmat Erwin Abdullah from Indonesia win a bronze medal lifting in the B group. In 2016 North Korean B group lifter Om Yun-chol won a gold medal and set an Olympic record in the clean and jerk. North Korean lifter Kim Myong-hyok, Poland's Tomasz Zieliński, and Cameroon's Madias Nzesso earned a silver out of the B group in 2012. And in 2004 B groups saw medals earned by Venezuela's Israel José Rubio and Belarus's Andrei Rybakou.

[17] All references to Daedelus and Icarus are taken from Ovid's *Metamorphosis*, Book VIII, 183-235.

[18] *Cratylus* 385

[19] *Cratylus* 390d

[20] *Cratylus* 435b

[21] *Cratylus* 435c

---

[22] *Cratylus* 385d-e

[23] *Cratylus* 386

[24] *Cratylus* 386e

[25] *Cratylus* 387

[26] *Cratylus* 387b

[27] *Cratylus* 389c

[28] Ibid. This theory, focused on a philosophy of language, later developed into Plato's Theory of Forms, is discussed in more detail in the chapter "On Perfection: Platonism and Competition."

[29] Calhoon G, Fry AC. Injury rates and profiles of elite competitive weightlifters. J Athl Train. 1999 Jul;34(3):232-8. PMID: 16558570; PMCID: PMC1322916.

[30] Ibid.

[31] Junge A, Engebretsen L, Mountjoy ML, Alonso JM, Renström PA, Aubry MJ, Dvorak J. Sports injuries during the Summer Olympic Games 2008. Am J Sports Med. 2009 Nov;37(11):2165-72. doi: 10.1177/0363546509339357. Epub 2009 Sep 25. PMID: 19783812.

[32] Perhaps an injury data set that will probably never be able to be accurately studied or reported is the frequency of various injuries across percentages of maximums, time into training sessions in which acute injuries occurred, and rates of injury recurrence across all age groups. Such a study might shed light on a few things. Percentage of maximums at which an injury either occurred or presented might tell us the role intensity plays in injury rates and severity. Time into training sessions might tell us whether an athlete is more likely to suffer an injury earlier in a training session (perhaps due to ineffective warm-up) or later in a training session (perhaps due to muscle fatigue or exhaustion affecting proper technique). And rates of recurrence across age groups would help clarify whether certain types of athletes are more or less prone to acute or chronic injury.

These studies, while enlightening, also do not appear to report the activity being performed when an injury occurs or presents itself. Specifically in the case of weightlifting, the amount of accessory work that occurs during training session is substantial enough that the injuries may occur or present themselves significantly more frequently during an accessory movement—e.g., back squatting, push pressing, etc.—than during the Olympic movements themselves—e.g., the snatch or the clean and jerk. If that is the case, then we can probably deduce that Olympic weightlifting is actually much safer than most other sports, at least on a non-Olympic level.

[33] This medal count reflects the gold, silver, and bronze medals awarded for the snatch and clean and jerk total. The World Weightlifting Championship also awarded medals for the best snatch and best clean and jerk.

[34] Epictetus, *Discourses* Book I, Chapter I

[35] Epictetus, *Discourses* Book I, Chapter III

[36] *Laches* 185d-186

[37] For more on this division of duties and the idea of a coach as a performer, see the chapter "On Coaching as a Performance: Aristotelian Categoriae."

[38] *Sophist* 240d To give Sophism a fair accounting, as Bertrand Russell reminds us in his *History of Western Philosophy*, "The word 'Sophist' had originally no bad connotation; it meat, as nearly as may be, what we mean by 'professor.'" Where there was no public education during the time of the Sophists, the group catered their teachings exclusively to young men with the means to pay for private instruction. Russell goes on to suggest that Plato's comfortable economic situation allowed him to occupy the latter of two camps: one with whom the Sophists were popular instructors and another who vilified the for-profit tutors as "frivolous and immoral."

[39] *Phaedrus* 265d

[40] Ibid.

[41] Ibid.

[42] *Philebus* 12e

[43] *Philebus* 12e-13

[44] *Sophist* 242-b

[45] Matthew 7:15 (KJV) can be credited with the introduction of the exact term *false prophet* and Mark 13:5-7 with a strikingly similar example of the difficulty of determining which prophets are false and which are true: "And Jesus answering them began to say, Take heed lest any *man* deceive you: For many shall come in my name, saying, I am *Christ*; and shall deceive many. And when ye shall hear of wars and rumours of wars, be ye not troubled: for *such things* must needs be; but the end *shall* not *be* yet."

[46] The collection of Aristotle's logical treatises is contained in six books referred to the Organon: *Categoriae* (Categories), *De Interpretatione* (On Interpretation), *Analytica Priora* (Prior Analytics), *Analytica Posteriora* (Posterior Analytics), *Topica* (Topics), and *De Sophisticis Elenchis* (On Sophistical Refutations).

[47] Elea was a town in Southern Italy known as the home of two of pre-Socratic history's most famous philosophers, Parmenides and Zeno.

[48] *Sophist* 240-240c

[49] *Sophist* 240d

[50] *Sophist* 242-b

[51] Durant, Will, *The Story of Philosophy*, p.9

[52] In *Sophist* 242c-243b, Theaetetus himself immediately waives this concern when the visitor offers up for critical examination the modes of instruction of famous pre-Socratics like Parmenides, Heraclitus, and Xenophanes. The visitor relates that it is "hard to say whether any one of these thinkers has told us the truth or not, and it wouldn't be appropriate for us to be critical of such renowned and venerable men." The problem with even these most venerable philosophers is that they do nothing more than explain without ensuring their students are learning. This difference, while subtle, is everything. For the visitor it is not enough that a teacher offers truths and goodness where the sophist offers deception if the truth-offeror is simply "talking their way through their explanations, without paying any attention to whether we were following them or were left behind." For more on this, see the chapter "On Selecting a Coach: The Systemic Art of Identifying the Sophist."

[53] Frg. 91 (Diels-Kranz)

[54] The Greek *ōsia* used here by Socrates refers to the Greek term for a thing or being's substance or essence. Other Greek terms in Socrates' dialectic have been omitted for clarity.

[55] *Cratylus* 401d

[56] Plutarch's Lives, Vol. 1, p. 13-14

[57] Harding, Phillip, *The Story of Athens: The Fragments of the Local Chronicles of Attika*, Harding estimates Theseus to have reigned from 1234 BC to 1205 BC.

[58] The underlying questions raised by the Ship of Theseus thought experiment lend themselves relatively simply to similar versions of the same puzzle with different philosophical questions. In 1655, a millennium and a half after Plutarch died, English political philosopher Thomas Hobbes asked whether, if all of the rotted planks were gathered up and put back together, the reassembled ship could also be called the Ship of Theseus. Hobbes, Thomas, *De Corpore*, ch 11.7

[59] *Parmenides* 139-b

[60] Frg. 91 (Diels-Kranz)

[61] Frg. 8 (Diels-Kranz)

[62] Frg. 8.26 (Diels-Kranz)

[63] *Parmenides* 127

[64] *Parmenides* 128

[65] *Parmenides* 128c-d

[66] Frg. 8.5-6 (Diels-Kranz)

[67] *Physics* VI.9, 239b5-7

[68] *Physics* VI.9, 239b12-13

[69] *Physics* VI.9, 239b15-18

[70] *Physics* VI.9, 239b8-9

[71] *Physics* VI.2, 233a22-32

[72] Laërtius, Diogenes, *Lives of the Eminent Philosophers*, vi. 39

[73] See *Plato: Complete Works*, Hackett ed, edited by John M. Copper and the Loeb Classical Library introduction to the Greater Hippias for two concise and somewhat opposing positions on Plato's authorship of *Hippias Major*.

[74] *Plato: Complete Works*, Hackett ed, edited by John M. Cooper.

[75] *Symposium* 211

[76] *Phaedo* 65d. For consistency's sake we will use the capitalized *Beauty* when referring to that attribute that beautiful things share and the lowercase *beauty* or *beautiful* when referring to that which is beautiful.

[77] *Cratylus* 440b

[78] *Greater Hippias* 287e

[79] *Greater Hippias* 289c

[80] *Greater Hippias* 289d-e

[81] *Greater Hippias* 291c

[82] *Greater Hippias* 291b

[83] *Greater Hippias* 295c

[84] *Greater Hippias* 296d-e

[85] For more on this part of the discussion begin at 298e where Socrates and Hippias agree that, while beautiful things are those that can be seen and heard, there are additional things that are beautiful that cannot be seen and heard such as delicious foods and sexual pleasure.

[86] Epictetus, *Discourses* Book I, Chapter VI

[87] Rules at that time required a 5kg jump between a lifter's first and second attempt. If a 2.5kg jump was made between the first and second attempts the lifter was denied a third attempt. However, if a competitor was within 10kg of the world record in the snatch or the clean and jerk, the lifter was permitted a fourth attempt so long as the attempt would set a new world record. And that fourth attempt only had to best the current record by 0.5kg. Pisarenko, of course, could have clean and jerked any weight above 265kg to secure the gold as well.

[88] For more on this see the chapter "On Perfection: Platonism and Competition."

[89] *Greater Hippias* 304e

[90] Throughout this chapter we will use the capitalized *Skeptic* to refer to the philosophers belonging to the ancient Greek school of Skepticism. This use should be distinguished from the more common *skeptic* which refers to those who are generally skeptical; those who have "doubts that a claim or statement is true or that something will happen." (Oxford Learner's Dictionary).

[91] Gorgias's writings have been lost to history so what we do know of them comes from commentaries by philosophers who lived over a half millennium after Gorgias died. *See* Sextus Empiricus *Against the Logicians* for an account of Gorgias's *On Non-Existence*. Professor Bruce McComiskey provides a concise treatment of *On Non-Existence* in "Gorgias, *On Non-Existence*: Sextus Empiricus, *Against the Logicians*" I.65-87, Translated from the Greek Text in Hermann Diels's *Die Fragmente der Vorsokratiker*."

[92] Russell, Bertrand, *The History of Western Philosophy*, p.233.

[93] Quoted in WARREN, J. (2000). ARISTOCLES' REFUTATIONS OF PYRRHONISM (Eus.PE 14.18.1-10). *Proceedings of the Cambridge Philological Society*, *46*, 140–164. http://www.jstor.org/stable/44696762. Warren carefully critiques Pyrrho's proposition that all things are indifferent: "On the manuscript reading we have no evidence of *why* all things are 'indifferent'. This is left simply as a grand metaphysical pronouncement in answer to the first of Timon's questions: 'How are things by nature?' But similarly with the emended text the Pyrrhonians have some argumentative work to do in order to sustain the claim about the unreliability of our senses and opinions."

[94] From the Stanford Encyclopedia of Philosophy: "The term 'epistemology' comes from the Greek words 'episteme' and 'logos'. 'Episteme' can be translated as 'knowledge' or 'understanding' or 'acquaintance', while 'logos' can be translated as 'account' or 'argument' or 'reason'." https://plato.stanford.edu/entries/epistemology/

[95] Quoted in WARREN, J. (2000). ARISTOCLES' REFUTATIONS OF PYRRHONISM (Eus.PE 14.18.1-10). *Proceedings of the Cambridge Philological Society*, *46*, 140–164.

[96] Ibid.

[97] Russell, Bertrand, *The History of Western Philosophy*, p.233. Russell also says of skepticism that it "was a lazy man's consolation, since it showed the ignorant to be as wise as the reputed

men of learning...it recommended itself as an antidote to worry" and, because of this, "Skepticism enjoyed a considerable popular success." at 234.

[98] *Metaphysica* I.1, 980a

[99] *Metaphysica* I.1, 980a

[100] Epicurus, *Principal Doctrines*, 24. Epicurus's full quote deserves reading here: "If you reject absolutely any single sensation without stopping to discriminate with respect to that which awaits confirmation between matter of opinion and that which is already present, whether in sensation or in feelings or in any immediate perception of the mind, you will throw into confusion even the rest of your sensations by your groundless belief and so you will be rejecting the standard of truth altogether. If in your ideas based upon opinion you hastily affirm as true all that awaits confirmation as well as that which does not, you will not escape error, as you will be maintaining complete ambiguity whenever it is a case of judging between right and wrong opinion."

We must therefore carefully word our call and response that "Epicurus *might respond to...*" because, as Professor Warren instructs in ARISTOCLES' REFUTATIONS OF PYRRHONISM, "Epicurus...and the early Epicureans show no knowledge of Pyrrho as an epistemologist...there is no evidence...that Pyrrho or the Pyrrhonians were one of the Epicureans' targets. The attacks on skepticism which can be found in Epicurean texts are generally thought to be aimed at Democriteanism." at 145.

[101] *Metaphysica* IV.5, 1010a1-4

[102] Quoted in WARREN, J. (2000). ARISTOCLES' REFUTATIONS OF PYRRHONISM (Eus.PE 14.18.1-10). *Proceedings of the Cambridge Philological Society, 46*, 140–164.

[103] *Analytica Posteriora* I.3, 72b5-6

[104] *Analytica Posteriora* I.3, 72b5-11

[105] *Analytica Posteriora* I.3, 72b12-13 This unknowability argument is known as *infinite regress*. Infinite regress is demonstrated as proposition $P1$ being questioned, answered, and then responded to by questioning $P2$ and so on. Think of any three-year-old child continually asking *but why* when given any normally satisfactory answer to the simplest of questions. That is a rough example of infinite regress.

[106] *Analytica Posteriora* I.3, 72b15-17

[107] Fragment 55: DK 22B55 In a later fragment Heraclitus admitted the danger of uninformed empiricism—overreliance on our senses without rational interpretation of what our senses tell us— "Eyes and ears are bad witnesses for men, since their souls lack understanding." Fragment 107: DK 22B107.

[108] *Metaphysica* I.3, 983a24-26

[109] *De Anima* III.8, 432a6-8

[110] *Metaphysica* IV.5, 1010b1-2

[111] *Metaphysica* IV.5, 1010b2-4

[112] Sextus *PH* 1.15 Regardless of what side of the sense and judgment argument one falls on, the Skeptics at least artfully followed their arguments to their logical conclusions however absurd and counterintuitive modern readers might find them. A later treatise by one Skeptic

explains that the philosophy follows "in practice the way of the world, but without holding any opinion of it." See Bevan, Edwyn, *Later Greek Religion*.

[113] *Analytica Priora* I.1, 24b18-20

[114] Tinkering around with Aristotelian syllogisms allows us to broaden some hypotheses to the point of absurdity. For example: All men are weak. Aristotle is a man. Aristotle is weak. The major and minor premises may coherently describe some state of the world, but the conclusion, while logically valid according to the premises, is not sound. For a fuller treatment on syllogisms and syllogistic fallacies and how some syllogistic problems can be solved, see Russinoff, I. S. (1999). The Syllogism's Final Solution. *The Bulletin of Symbolic Logic*, 5(4), 451–469. https://doi.org/10.2307/421118.

[115] Aristotle offers a neater definition than our *loosely formulated piece of logic* saying, "I call that a perfect syllogism which needs nothing other than what has been stated to make plain what necessarily follows." *Analytica Priora* I.1, 24b23-24

[116] *Rhetorica* I.1, 1354a14-15

[117] *Analytica Priora* II 70a9-10

[118] *Analytica Priora* Bk II 70a3-5, 6-7

[119] *Analytica Priora* Bk I 24b

[120] *Analytica Priora* Bk I Ch I 24b20-25

[121] *Analytica Priora* I.5,.27a5

[122] *De Sophisticis Elenchis* 5 166b28: note that the use of the term *accident* in philosophy is importantly distinct from its common usage. Whereas in today's language *accident* is generally understood to mean some sort of unintended mistake or blunder, in philosophy it simply means that which is not necessarily so.

[123] *De Sophisticis Elenchis* 5 166b28

[124] Laërtius, Diogenes, *Lives of the Eminent Philosophers*, iii. 46

[125] *Politics* V.10, 1311b20-2

[126] https://olympics.com/en/athletes/leonid-zhabotinsky

[127] https://olympics.com/en/athletes/waldemar-baszanowski

[128] Keeping in mind that *body* does not necessarily mean a human body Aristotle seems to put *body* in both *substance* (*Categoriae* 3a) and *quantity* (*Categoriae* 5a).

[129] At least with regard to the genomically sequenced 4th century Stagirite Aristotle.

[130] *Categoriae* 7

[131] *Categoriae* 6b20-25

[132] *Categoriae* 8b25

[133] *Categoriae* 8b27-9a

[134] *Categoriae* 9a13-25 Aristotle's argument for healthiness and sickliness being an inborn capacity rests on his claim that "men are called healthy in virtue of the inborn capacity of easy resistance to those unhealthy influences that may ordinarily arise; unhealthy, in virtue of the lack of this capacity."

[135] *Categoriae* 9a28-32

[136] *Categoriae* 10a10-15

[137] *Categoriae* 10a25

138 *Categoriae* 10b25

139 *Categoriae* 1a

140 *Categoriae* 1a6

141https://www.teamusa.org/USA-Weightlifting/Features/2021/August/02/Sarah-Robles-Becomes-First-US-Woman-to-Win-Two-Olympic-Weightlifting-Medals

142https://www.teamusa.org/USA-Weightlifting/Features/2022/January/19/USA-Weightlifting-Expands-High-Performance-Division-With-New-Team-Members

143 *Categoriae* 10b25

144 https://olympics.com/en/athletes/pyrros-dimas

145 See the chapter "On Perfection: Platonism and Competition."

146 A teaching advantage is simply that which gives some teacher some edge over another teacher. For example, an ability to impart knowledge better than some other coach, the ability to understand the right type of motivation to the right athlete at the right time, or the ability to recognize in her clients some adaptability to some movement or set or rep scheme that is easily expounded to the benefit of both coach and athlete.

147 *Republic III* 411d

148 *Republic III* 410

149 *Republic III* 410d